More Fat-Burning Foods

More
Fat-
Burning
Foods

and Other Weight-Loss Secrets

Porter Shimer

Recipes edited by Betty Bianconi, R.D.

CB

CONTEMPORARY BOOKS

Library of Congress Cataloging-in-Publication Data

Shimer, Porter.
    More fat-burning foods and other weight-loss secrets / Porter Shimer :
recipes edited by Betty Bianconi.
            p.   cm.
    Originally published: Owings Mills, Md. : Ottenheimer Publishers, 1998.
    ISBN 0-8092-2599-9
    1. Reducing diets.   2. Weight loss.   I. Bianconi, Betty.   II. Title.
RM222.2.S527   1998
613.2'5—dc21   99-12083
                                                                            CIP

Originally published by Ottenheimer Publishers, Inc.

This editiion first published in 1999 by Contemporary Books
A division of NTC/Contemporary Publishing Group, Inc.
4255 West Touhy Avenue, Lincolnwood (Chicago), Illinois 60646-1975 U.S.A.
Printed in the United States of America
International Standard Book Number: 0-8092-2599-9
18   17   16   15   14   13   12   11   10   9   8   7   6   5   4   3   2   1

CONTENTS

INTRODUCTION

Hello—and welcome to the end of your struggles to lose weight.

No matter how many times you have tried before, this time you're going to succeed! The reason: You're going to learn how to live *with* food rather than without it.

If food was your enemy before, it will soon be your friend. No longer will you fear it, or feel guilty about eating it, or have to endure the pain of doing without it. The truth is, the fatal flaw of your previous weight-loss efforts probably has been that you've been trying to eat too little!

No way, you say? It's those second helpings and midnight trips to the refrigerator that are your downfall?

Well, while it's true that those activities certainly won't help you lose weight, have you ever asked yourself why you feel the need for that extra food? Hunger, perhaps? Feelings of deprivation? Or could your body be telling you that it's not happy skipping breakfast, or eating just a salad for lunch, or pouring "dinner" from an eight-ounce can?

Fact: Any weight-loss effort that deprives us is going to fail. That's a rule engraved in the very genes that have gotten us where we are today. Our ancestors who lived in caves survived because they were able to feed their hunger, not ignore it. Why should we be any different?

We aren't, as the latest surveys make painfully clear. During the past 40 years, when "dieting" has become so popular, we've not only not lost weight, we've gained an average of 10 pounds. That's right: We're fatter today than we were back when we buttered our white bread clear to the edges, went to the malt shop instead of the gym, and ate our cheeseburgers guilt-free!

The "Dieter's" Dilemma

Our diets have failed not just because they ask us to accept feeling hungry but because they undermine the very biochemical processes on which fat-loss depends. Studies now show that to burn fat most effectively, our bodies need energy—something that's in very short supply when dinner is little more than a salad or a cup of broth. Think of the excess fat on your body as something like a log in a fireplace: Without energy from the right "kindling"—that is, food—your body cannot generate enough heat to get the fat "burning" as energy.

In fact, the less we eat, the more stubborn our body fat becomes. This is because cutting calories forces our bodies into what scientists call their "starvation response"—a holdover from prehistoric times when we learned to burn fewer calories as a way of preserving body fat to help us survive times of famine. The consequence of this response for us today, unfortunately, is that the fewer calories we consume, the more inclined our bodies are to store these calories as fat.

Making matters even worse is what low-calorie diets do to our metabolism in the long run: By causing the loss of muscle tissue, which is the best calorie burner we have, diets make us even more prone to gain weight when the diet is over.

The end result is a "Catch-22" you may know all too well. You are haunted by hunger pangs and cravings when you're on a low-calorie diet, and whatever you do eat becomes even more fattening because your metabolism has slowed to a crawl. Worse yet, *you* slow to a crawl. Out of calories and "out of gas," you're left with barely enough energy to go about your day. You certainly don't feel like engaging in any fat-burning or muscle-building exercises.

Fat-Burning Foods to the Rescue

There is a solution to the dilemma—and it's a surprisingly simple and appetizing one: To keep your fat-burning fires adequately "stoked," you've got to eat!

But before you call your local pizzeria or head to the nearest ice cream parlor, be aware that you can't eat just anything you want. If you fill up on foods that are high in fat or that contain too much refined sugar, you'll be feeding your fat cells instead of starving them. What you will have to do is stoke your body's fat-burning fires with the foods it will use directly and immediately for energy.

We'll be looking at these foods and the biology behind their fat-burning powers shortly, but let it suffice to say that not all foods are created equal when it comes to weight gain. Calorie-for-calorie, some foods are better at burning fat while others are more chemically suited for becoming fat. A lifetime of successful weight control, therefore, can become a simple matter of consuming more of the former foods and less of the latter.

Fat-Burning for the Health of It

Weight control aside, there's another reason fat-burning foods should be on your table every day: They can be your "meal ticket" to better health. Studies by such prestigious organizations as the American Heart Association, the American Cancer Society, and the Centers for Disease Control and Prevention in Atlanta now show that a diet centered around these foods can help reduce risks of virtually every major illness we face today, including heart disease, high blood pressure, strokes, diabetes, osteoporosis (softening of the bones), and cancers of the prostate, cervix, and breast.

That these foods also are economical and among the most tasty on the planet is simply icing on the cake.

At the end of this book, you will have learned about foods that will help you live not only leaner but longer! So make yourself comfortable and get ready to say goodbye to your fat.

Get ready, too, to learn about the right ways to exercise to give these foods an even greater fat-burning effect. Exercise— by bringing oxygen into the body like a strong breeze to a brush fire—has been shown to turn up the metabolic "heat" of fat-burning foods even more. Exercise also can help maintain and build the muscle tissue that is your body's greatest ally for making weight loss last.

Encouraged? Good. You should be. You're about to embark on the weight-loss venture that will be your last!

CHAPTER 1

YOUR FULL—AND
FLAT!—STOMACH

Have you ever noticed how your appetite can be like a bar of wet soap: The more you try to control it, the more it's apt to slip away? You can be good for a while, but then whammo: out come the butter pecan ice cream and the chocolate marshmallow cookies.

There's a reason for this, and it goes as far back as we do—back to when a full stomach was a goal and not a source of guilt. "Severe calorie restriction runs counter to a very basic human instinct," says Yale University psychologist Judith Roden, Ph.D., "which is to perceive hunger as a threat."

In other words, our aversion to hunger is in our genes. We endured the rigors of our evolution by eating what we could, when we could. Survival of the fittest meant survival of the fullest, and to a degree we are genetically programmed to think of food in these same terms today.

F.Y.I.

Number of Americans currently
   on a diet: 48 million

Percentage increase in overweight
   Americans over the past 10 years: 28

Weight the average American gains
   between the ages of 25 and 55:   30 pounds

Amount of muscle that converts to fat
   during this time: 15 pounds

Percentage of Americans who exercise
   irregularly or not at all: 58

Number one excuse given by the average
   American for not exercising more: Lack of time

Minutes per day the average American
   watches TV: 240

Estimated yearly cost associated with
   health complications caused by obesity: $68.8 billion

Diets Teach Fat to Fight Back

We go head-to-head with Mother Nature when we try to starve ourselves thin, and it's a battle Mother Nature wins nearly every time. As we saw in our introduction, severely restricting calories not only slows the rate at which our bodies burn calories, it robs us of the very muscle tissue on which fat-burning depends! This is why nine out of ten dieters who attempt to reduce their caloric intake fail.

Reducing calories is a trap that has snared dieters by the millions. In fact, many nutritionists feel that our attempts to lose weight have been a major reason we've put on so much weight. Low-calorie diets teach our bodies to hold on to the very fat we're trying so desperately to lose.

"Diets teach fat cells to defend themselves," explains nutritionist Debrah Waterhouse. "Fat cells evolved to keep us alive during times of famine, and they interpret low-calorie diets as just that—a famine. They respond by holding onto the fat they already have, and by becoming even more aggressive at taking in new fat once the diet is over. The result is a system of fat protection that can be very hard to break, especially since the system gets stronger each time a new diet is tried."

Eating Less But Weighing More

Now we understand that drastically cutting calories can actually make fat cells more stubborn. The average woman today, despite consuming 200 fewer calories a day, weighs six pounds more than the average woman did 30 years ago. Might it be because she has been on an average of ten diets in her lifetime?

Witness, moreover, the bodily "inflation" we've suffered in the last 10 years alone, a decade during which dieters have joined weight-loss programs in record numbers. The National Center for Health Statistics reports that while 41 percent of women and 51 percent of men exceeded acceptable weight limits in 1987, both of those figures are up by nearly 20 percent today.

Dieting is so damaging to the body's ability to burn fat, some doctors actually put their underweight patients on low-calorie diets, followed by periods of normal eating, to give their bodies a fat-gaining boost!

Weighty Matters

Average yearly cost of participating in a
   commercial weight-loss program: $608

Number of people participating in
commercial weight-loss programs
who maintain their weight loss for
at least seven years: One out of 250

Average cost of liposuction
   (surgical removal of fat): $5,000 per pound!

Percentage of liposuction patients
who experience a regrowth of
their fat: 29

Satisfaction Guaranteed

Are you afraid that hunger might be a problem on a low-fat diet? Then feast on this fact. To get the same amount of fat in just one fast-food super burger, such as a Whopper or a Big Mac (approximately 60 grams), you would have to eat all of the following:

- *half a pound of broiled chicken*
- *four ounces of a low-fat fish*
- *six scallops*
- *an entire head of lettuce*
- *one onion*
- *one cup of kidney beans*
- *one cup of brown rice*
- *one pound of string beans*
- *one sweet potato*
- *one ear of sweet corn*
- *one cup of raisins*
- *one orange*
- *two red beets*
- *four spears of asparagus*
- *one half pound of peas*
- *one cup of air-popped popcorn*
- *one cup of cooked spaghetti*
- *two slices of whole wheat bread*

Now that's a sandwich!

Race Not Always to the Swift

Wait a minute? No miraculous overnight results? You were hoping to squeeze into that size eight by the weekend?

Sorry, but fat loss—true fat loss—cannot be rushed. Most experts now agree that losses of approximately one pound a week are best to assure that the majority of the weight lost will be from actual fat. Any diet that has you losing weight faster than that is going to be cheating you in either of two ways: It's going to have you losing mere water weight, which you can gain back with one trip to the water cooler, or it's going to cost you the muscle tissue needed to make your weight loss last.

Sure, when you lose weight fast, you can weigh less according to your bathroom scale. But not because you've actually lost any appreciable amounts of fat and not because you've done anything to improve your chances of maintaining a desirable weight in the future. There's a rule of thumb regarding weight loss in this regard that you might consider posting on your refrigerator door:

The Longer Weight Loss Takes, The Longer It's Going To Last!

Losing weight is a race won by the tortoise rather than the hare. You've got to learn to get comfortable with the foods that are not just going to get you thinner, but that will keep you that way for the rest of your life.

Fat-Burning Foods under the Microscope

And just what sort of foods might these be? Lots of lettuce and celery, perhaps? There's certainly not a lot of fat-making potential there, right? Or will it be some bizarre combination like vinegar and ice cream? (Now there's a combo sure to limit your caloric intake!)

Relax. Not only are the best foods for burning fat surprisingly "normal," they are tasty, nutritious, and filling. They're foods you see in your supermarket every time you shop. If there's anything "unusual" about these foods, it's that they have a biochemical inclination for helping your body get rid of fat rather than store it. They're fat "breakers" not fat "makers."

FAT-BURNING FACT:

Percentage of people able to stop taking high blood pressure medication after losing just 10 pounds: 60.

If that sounds a little too good to be true, it's not. Research shows that certain foods, with one or more of the following components, are capable of waging war against fat:

• **Complex Carbohydrates:** Capable of fighting fat by providing the energy needed to step up the body's basic metabolic (fat-burning) rate. Complex carbohydrates are found in starchy foods such as breads, potatoes, cereals, pasta, and rice. They are not to be confused with the faster-digested simple carbohydrates (sucrose, glucose, and fructose) found in sweet-tasting foods such as candies, cookies, soft drinks, and sugary desserts. Because simple carbohydrates contain virtually no nutrients or fiber, and because they fail to provide feelings of fullness as complex carbohydrates do, they should be eaten sparingly as part of a fat-burning diet.

• **Fiber:** Capable of fighting fat by controlling insulin levels (and hence the ease with which calories can be stored as fat) and by providing feelings of fullness. Fiber also helps to send fats through the intestines before they have time to be fully absorbed. Fiber is most abundant in fruits, vegetables, beans, and whole-grain cereals and breads.

• **Low-Fat Protein:** Capable of fighting fat by building and maintaining fat-burning muscle tissue and by preventing other foods (including carbohydrates) from being digested too quickly. Best sources are low-fat varieties of fish and seafood, lean meats, low-fat dairy products, and beans.

• **Healthful Fats:** Capable of fighting fat by providing feelings of fullness and by controlling cravings. Research also shows that healthful fats—the monounsaturated fat found in olive oil, for example, and the polyunsaturated omega-3 fatty acids found in fish—can help keep the heart and blood vessels healthy by lowering levels of harmful (LDL) cholesterol in the blood. The type of fat to avoid is the saturated fat found in beef, pork, the skin of chicken and turkey, and full-fat dairy products such as whole milk, ice cream, and cheese.

Your Top Fat-Burning Foods

The following types of foods should make up the bulk of your diet if you're really serious about achieving and maintaining a healthy weight for the rest of your life. The list is by no means complete. Many other fruits, vegetables, complex carbohydrates, and low-fat proteins also can act as valuable weight-control allies. Consider this list of foods as a foundation for getting your lifelong weight-control program off to a healthful—and delicious!—start.

Fruits	Vegetables	Complex Carbohydrates	Low-Fat Proteins
Apples	Asparagus	Bagels	Chicken breast
Blueberries	Beets	Beans (all types)	Egg whites*
Citrus fruits	Broccoli	Couscous	Low-fat cottage cheese
Kiwi fruit	Brussels sprouts	Oatmeal	Low-fat fish
Melons	Carrots	Pasta	Low-fat yogurt
Peaches	Eggplant	Rice	White meat turkey
Strawberries	Green beans	Whole-grain breads	
	Onions		
	Potatoes		
	Yams		* or non-fat egg substitutes

The Importance of Balance

Potatoes! Pasta! Bagels! You'll be in high-carbohydrate heaven!

But wait! Let's not forget that your ideal fat-burning diet should be a balance of these fat-burning foods. Don't make the mistake of concentrating too heavily on one type. That could be the reason past weight-loss programs have failed. Diets that focus too narrowly on a single food group miss the forest for the trees, sacrificing health and/or flavor along the way.

High-protein diets, for example, achieve weight loss primarily through reducing the water in your body, and diets that allow only limited types of foods (the "ice cream diet" or the "grapefruit diet") usually wind up being simply low-calorie regimens because the monotony of the menu causes dieters to lose their appetites. Even diets too high in otherwise healthful carbohydrates can backfire by causing high levels of insulin in the blood, which results in seemingly insatiable hunger.

Not so if you eat the right foods in the right balance. Most nutritionists now agree that the most healthful diet consists of the following:

- 60 percent of calories from carbohydrates (preferably complex)

- 15 percent from protein

- 25 percent from fat (no more than 10 percent saturated)

FOOD GUIDE PYRAMID

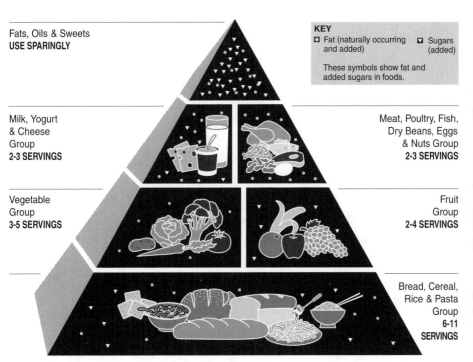

Fats, Oils & Sweets
USE SPARINGLY

KEY
☐ Fat (naturally occurring and added)   ☑ Sugars (added)

These symbols show fat and added sugars in foods.

Milk, Yogurt
& Cheese
Group
2-3 SERVINGS

Meat, Poultry, Fish,
Dry Beans, Eggs
& Nuts Group
2-3 SERVINGS

Vegetable
Group
3-5 SERVINGS

Fruit
Group
2-4 SERVINGS

Bread, Cereal,
Rice & Pasta
Group
**6-11
SERVINGS**

Source: U.S. Department of Agriculture/U.S. Department of Health and Human Services

21

Climb the Food Pyramid to Better Health

If those numbers confuse you, take a look at the food "pyramid" on the previous page. It was created by the U.S. Department of Agriculture (USDA) to make it easier for Americans to get a clearer "picture" of what a healthful diet should include.

Grain-based Foods *(6 to 11 servings daily):* This is the food group that should make up the bulk of your diet. It includes breads, rice, cereals, and pastas—all important for adding fat-burning complex carbohydrates to your diet.

Fruits *(2 to 4 servings)* **and Vegetables** *(3 to 5 servings):* This is the second most important food group. It is vital for adding important vitamins, minerals, and fiber to your diet.

Protein Foods—Dairy Products *(2 to 3 servings)* **and Meats, Beans, and Eggs** *(2 to 3 servings):* This group makes up the third level of the pyramid. Protein foods are important for maintaining healthy muscle tissue—the best fat-burning tissue your body has.

Fats and Sweets: This is the least important food group and includes butter, margarine, cooking oils, and foods high in refined sugar such as candies and rich desserts. Foods from this group should be eaten sparingly.

Some Facts About Fat
A Fair Shake for Fat: A Little Dab Will Do

But what is any kind of fat doing on a weight-loss program? Doesn't that stuff serve up nine calories per gram compared with only four for carbohydrates and proteins? And isn't fat a major cause of heart disease? And hasn't new research shown that fat's calories are actually more fattening than those from carbohydrates or proteins because, once digested, they turn more easily into fat?

Yes to all of the above. But that doesn't mean that limited amounts of the right kinds of fat can't help grease the wheels of a successful weight-loss program. Research now shows that certain amounts of fat may be needed to slow the rate at which carbohydrates are metabolized. This helps put the brakes on hunger. In fact, some fats are now being recognized as actually lowering cholesterol levels in the blood, which is good for the blood vessels and the heart.

Learn What Kinds of Fat You're up Against

Before you refill your butter dish, understand that we're not talking about a lot of fat—approximately 25 percent of total calories—and that not all types of fat are worthy of inclusion. The most healthful fats are monounsaturated and polyunsaturated fats (for best sources, see below). The fats to avoid are saturated fats, which are found principally in full-fat dairy products, such as butter, and in hydrogenated oils, beef, and pork. Studies show that these fats, in addition to piling on the calories, are without a doubt the primary contributors to the build-up of LDL cholesterol (the bad kind) and other fatty substances in the blood.

As proof, witness one study that found no decreases in cholesterol levels for people on a diet that contained just 25 percent fat but all of it saturated. When these same people were switched to a low-fat diet with unsaturated fat, their cholesterol levels quickly fell by an average of 20 percent.

But cholesterol aside, all fats, regardless of type, are high in calories (approximately 120 calories per tablespoon). Therefore they should be consumed sparingly as part of your fat-burning diet. Keep that in mind as you make that oil and vinegar salad dressing, or prepare to sauté vegetables. Whether it's "good" or "bad" oil, use as little as possible!

FAT-BURNING FACT:

Studies show that for every one percent drop in serum cholesterol levels, the risk of heart disease drops by two percent.

Good Fats
Monounsaturated:

Olive oil	(75%)*
Canola oil	(60%)
Peanut oil	(50%)

In Between Fats
Polyunsaturated:

Safflower oil	(75%)
Sunflower oil	(70%)
Corn oil	(60%)
Cottonseed oil	(55%)

Bad Fats
Saturated:

Coconut oil	(90%)
Butter fat	(65%)
Beef fat	(50%)
Palm oil	(50%)
Chicken fat	(30%)

----

*Percentages refer to the amount that each oil or fat is comprised of the type of fat represented.

Why Fat Is So Fattening

But please don't be lulled into a sense of false security about the advisability of a certain amount of fat in your weight-control plans. Given our current average intake (approximately 38 percent of calories according to most estimates), the fat in our diets remains the number one contributor to the fat on our bodies. Until we accept that fact—and do something about it—our best weight-loss efforts are going to be exercises in futility.

If your diet is like most people's, you're going to have to cut back on fat to encourage your body to burn more fat. (You may consider that another cardinal rule of weight loss worthy of being displayed prominently on your refrigerator door!)

Why Is Fat Such a Dieter's Waterloo?

Because in addition to containing more than twice as many calories as carbohydrates and proteins per gram, food fat becomes body fat quite easily. While carbohydrates and proteins require considerable "work" from our digestive systems before they are converted to body fat, food fat turns into body fat quickly and easily—within hours of ingestion, in fact. The reason, not surprisingly, is that dietary fat and body fat are chemically very similar. Therefore, very few biochemical steps are needed to make the dietary fat to body fat conversion.

Not so with carbohydrates and proteins. Studies show that nearly one quarter of the calories from carbohydrates and proteins go directly to revving up the body's fat-burning engines. The rest will be stored for later use.

Consider, for example, the following numbers: If you were to eat 100 calories from fat, only 3 of those calories would boost your body's metabolic (calorie-burning) rate. But eat 100 calories in the form of carbohydrates or proteins and whammo: 23 of those calories go toward stoking your body's fat-burning fires.

Fat Really Does "Stick to the Ribs"

If that sounds like much ado about nothing, it's not. A difference of 23 calories for every 100 calories consumed can begin to add up quickly, as people taking part in a study reported in the *International Journal of Obesity* several years ago found out. The people were put on one of two very high-calorie diets—one high in fat, the other low in fat but high in carbohydrates. The purpose of the experiment was to see if there might be a difference in how long it would take for people to gain weight on each diet. There was a difference—a huge one.

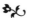

> "We need to start thinking of the fat we eat as the fat we wear."
>
> *Peter Vash, M.D, Professor of Medicine,*
> *University of California*

While the people on the low-fat diet took a little over seven months to gain 30 pounds, those assigned to the high-fat regimen amassed their 30 pounds in less than half that time, even though their diet was slightly lower in calories. (Not surprisingly, the people on the high-fat diet, more so than the low-fat group, gained weight primarily in the stomach area.)

So yes, the old saying that fatty foods "stick to the ribs" may be truer than we've known.

Trimming Fat Can Make "Cents," Too!

But aren't low-fat and calorie-reduced foods costly?

Yes, fat-reduced versions of some foods can be more expensive than their regular counterparts, but many foods that are naturally low in fat tend to be cheaper than fattier alternatives. Potatoes, beans, rice, and pasta are fantastic food bargains.

Researchers from Columbia University monitored the food costs of 291 people on low-fat diets for a period of nine months. The food bills of these people averaged approximately a dollar a day less on their low-fat regimens, which researchers calculated could save the average family of four approximately $1,000 dollars a year.

Now that's a nice bonus for eating healthfully. By thinning your waist, you fatten your wallet!

Less Fat for More Muscle

The process by which dietary fat becomes body fat is simple and direct because the two are chemically similar in the first place. Carbohydrates and low-fat proteins, by comparison, prefer not to be turned into fat at all. They're chemically more suited to being consumed by muscle cells for the production of energy. Better yet, some research has suggested that eating carbohydrates and low-fat proteins may encourage muscular growth even without additional exercise.

This was demonstrated in an experiment conducted by researchers from the University of Illinois in which women on low-fat, high-carbohydrate diets not only lost substantial amounts of body fat, they actually boosted their muscle mass by a surprising 2.2 percent. That might not sound like a lot, but the increase occurred without the women engaging in any exercise outside their normal routines. How was that muscle "born"?

The researchers speculated that the high-carbohydrate diet may have increased the women's energy levels to a point where they had become more active without realizing it!

Runners have been aware of the energizing effects of carbohydrates for years. Carbohydrates do well at fueling exercise because they turn into glucose, your body's favorite muscle fuel, so quickly after ingestion. Michael Yessis, Ph.D., exercise physiologist and author of *Body Shaping* (Rodale Press, 1993), puts it this way: "Carbohydrates make you feel most like exercising, they provide the best fuel for that exercise, and they do the best job of replenishing muscles with the fuels that exercise uses up."

Fat Cells: "Fitter" Than Muscle Cells for Regrowth

It doesn't seem fair, but it's a fact of life, nonetheless. While the number of muscle cells we have is fixed at birth (exercise can only make them larger; it cannot increase their number), fat cells can begin to split and multiply any time we eat enough to allow them to become "too big for their britches."

To make matters worse, "The number of fat cells we have can always go up, but never come down," says Dr. Glenn Gaesser, a professor of exercise physiology at the University of Virginia and the author of *Big Fat Lies* (Ballantine Books, 1996). "Once we've got them, they're ours to keep."

"Exercising with a friend gives many people a surge of energy on days when they otherwise wouldn't feel like working out."

Jonathan Robison, Ph.D., Executive Co-Director of the Michigan Center for Preventative Medicine

This is not the case with muscle cells, unfortunately, which can wither and die if we don't give them enough to do. This is why it is so important to avoid obesity, which is caused by overeating and lack of exercise. It trades muscle cells for fat cells in a "deal" that can never be fully undone.

The Satisfaction Factor

Okay, so a low-fat, high-carbohydrate diet can be great for providing energy and burning fat. But will such a diet be able to keep visions of cheesecake from dancing in our heads? There's not an apple on earth, after all, that can satisfy like a hot fudge sundae with jimmies.

Try telling that to the group of students who took part in an interesting study done recently at the University of Sydney in Australia. The students were asked to eat 240-calorie portions of dozens of different foods, after which they were measured for degrees of fullness at 15-minute intervals for a period of two hours. Much to everyone's amazement—including the students'—apples satisfied twice as long as ice cream. A bowl of oatmeal satisfied three times longer than a doughnut. A potato six times longer than a croissant.

So, no, foods do not have to be high in fat to satisfy. Other factors are more important. Things such as the sheer weight and volume of a particular food, which signal feelings of fullness within the digestive tract. And how long it takes to chew the food—the longer the better so that feelings of fullness can have time to occur before too many calories have been consumed. (How long, after all, does it take to scarf down a 400-calorie piece of cheesecake?) Critical, too, is the amount of fiber in the food. In addition to having the weight-control advantage of sweeping fats through the intestines undigested, fiber gives us a feeling of fullness by absorbing water.

Bottom line: Some of the best foods for weight loss also can be the most satisfying, and if you don't think so, just take a look at the following list. These are the foods that scored the highest, and the lowest, in the "satiation contest" mentioned above.

The numbers that follow these foods refer to the food's "satiation index," that is, the food's ability to quell hunger for as long, and for as few calories, as possible. (Incidentally, virtually all of the "best" foods appear prominently on the list of fat-burning foods that we recommend as the key players in your fat-burning diet!)

Foods To Fill You UP, Not OUT

Best:		Satiation Index
	Potatoes:	323
	Fish:	225
	Oatmeal:	209
	Oranges:	202
	Apples:	197
	Pasta (whole wheat):	188
	Lean beef:	176
	Grapes:	162
	Popcorn (air-popped):	154
	Bran cereal:	151
Worst:		
	Ice cream:	96
	Potato chips:	91
	Peanuts:	84
	Candy bar (chocolate):	70
	Doughnut:	68
	Cake:	65
	Croissant:	47

Getting Your Taste Buds in Shape

Low-fat foods can satisfy your stomach, but what about your taste buds? Won't a low-fat diet leave you craving the taste of high-fat foods even though your tummy might be content?

"People who switch to low-fat diets sometimes experience a short period of mild withdrawal in the beginning," says Bryant Stamford, Ph.D., director of the Center for Health Promotion at the University of Louisville, who recently overhauled his own less-than-lean diet. "But within several weeks, the body adjusts and people often find that fats actually become uncomfortable to digest because their bodies begin producing less fat-digesting enzymes. In my own case, the kind of breakfast I used to be able to eat without any problem now would leave me feeling quite ill."

FAT-BURNING FACT:

Percentage of people who have ever lied about their weight: 33.

The enzyme most responsible for the digestion of fats is called lipoprotein lipase (LPL), and it can work much to our disadvantage when we eat fats regularly, says Dr. Stamford. "This is because LPL helps break fats down into molecules small enough to be absorbed by fat cells, and the more fat we eat, unfortunately, the more active this enzyme becomes. Worse yet, this enzyme also becomes more active the fatter we become, so a doubly fattening momentum can begin to build when fatty foods become a regular part of a person's diet."

Sweets Double the Trouble

Worse yet, a preference for sweets can make the fat in our diets even more "fattening," Dr. Stamford explains, because sugar boosts the fat-storing power of LPL to an even higher level. "This is why most junk foods are such dietary disasters. They tend to contain both sugar and fat in very large amounts."

What this means is that junk foods not only swing the doors of fat cells wide open, they also assure that molecules of fat make themselves all-too comfortable once inside.

Try to stay away from particularly harmful "sweet and fatty" combinations to keep your fat-burning fires burning most brightly.

CAUTION: High Risk Area

Buttered toast with jam	Donuts
Cake	Ice cream (except low-fat or sugar-free)
Candy bars (most)	Pancakes or waffles with butter and syrup
Chocolate	Pastries
Cookies	Pies (fruit as well as custards)
Croissants (filled)	Puddings

Lower Fat, Higher Spirits

But let's face it, there's more to life than just a flat tummy. Will reducing the fat in your diet also reduce your fun? Will life without your favorite high-fat sweets turn sour?

Not if the conclusions of a recent study by the University of Washington in Seattle are any indication. That study monitored the moods of 555 women who cut the fat in their diets in half for a year. The women reported a significant lift in their spirits—and not just because they lost an average of nine pounds. In fact, they said they felt more energetic and upbeat than they had when "comforted" by their high-fat diets of old.

Why?

Feelings of accomplishment were a factor, no doubt, but some hard-core physiology may also have been at work. Studies show that eating less fat results in greater oxygen flow and hence more energy for every cell in the body, including those of the "mood center" we call the brain.

FAT-BURNING FACT:

Once a fat cell has been created, it cannot be destroyed. Muscle cells, on the other hand, will wither and die if not exercised adequately.

The Top Ten Reasons Dieters Fail

Why do nine out of ten dieters fail to maintain their weight loss for more than a few months, with many putting on even more weight when their diets are over? Weight-loss experts cite the following reasons:

1. **They bite off less than they can chew.** Reducing caloric intake to near starvation levels slows the fat-burning process on which long-term weight control depends. It also sets dieters up for binges, as it robs them of the energy needed for fat-burning exercise. For weight loss to be safe and effective, your diet should include no fewer than 1,200 calories a day.

2. **They lose too fast.** Any diet that produces rapid weight loss risks "throwing the baby out with the bath water." Such a diet reduces valuable calorie-burning muscle tissue, not just fat. Most experts agree on a weight loss of no more than one pound a week.

3. **They assume that all calories are created equal.** New research shows that calories from dietary fat convert more easily to body fat than calories from carbohydrates or protein. A diet high in fat can be "fattening," even though its caloric content may be relatively low.

4. **They break rather than bend.** Too often dieters allow minor slips to become major falls. "Just one" becomes more like one dozen. The key to permanent weight control is learning to be good, not perfect.

5. **They underestimate the value of exercise.** Not only is exercise a fantastic calorie burner while in progress, it can burn calories for as long as several hours afterward. It's also an effective muscle builder, appetite suppressant, and mood elevator and therefore deserves to be a daily "main course."

6. **They get out of "balance."** Relying too heavily on any one type of food to lose weight is shortsighted and potentially dangerous. Effective weight loss requires a healthy and energetic body, not a sick one.

7. **They aspire to the impossible.** No weight-loss effort in the world is going to alter basic body type. Any diet trying to convert a Rosie O'Donnell type into a Cindy Crawford is more likely to result in loss of self-esteem than weight.

8. **They lack support.** Losing weight is a tough enough job on your own; lack of support from family members and friends can make it even tougher. Studies show that chances for success increase with the support of loved ones and peers.

9. **They succumb to advertising.** It's a fattening world we live in, made even more so by the advertising expertise of the food industry. It's a fact that weight loss and frequent TV-watching make for a counterproductive relationship.

10. **They don't really try.** Sorry, but some studies suggest that real commitment may be one of the highest weight-loss hurdles of all. Millions of people say they want to lose weight, only to find that their stomachs speak louder than their hearts—and brains!

"Mind Games" for Taming Your Appetite

Yes, there are some ways to satisfy hunger that go beyond the stomach. Research shows that we can help put our appetites to rest by soothing our brains as well. Here are some hunger-taming "tricks" worth trying:

- *Dim the lights.* Studies by The Johns Hopkins University in Baltimore show that people tend to eat more in environments where lighting is bright and colors are vibrant. Try dimming the lights for your next evening meal, or go one better and break out the candles!

- *Dine from plainer plates.* Research shows, too, that plates with busy patterns tend to be appetite stimulants, so go plain, Jane. You might also want to switch to smaller plates, as they can trick our tummies into feeling fuller on less.

- *Develop a taste for tepid tunes.* The faster the music, the faster we eat, so make your stereo selections accordingly. Better to dine to Julio Iglesias than Nine Inch Nails. (Save your punk rock favorites for your exercise class.)

FAT-BURNING FACT:

There's more fat in a single teaspoon of butter than in 10 pounds of potatoes.

The Problems with Protein—and How to Solve Them

Where does protein fit into a fat-burning diet?

Intimately, but with one critical provision. While protein is essential to a fat-burning diet to maintain fat-burning muscle tissue, the protein must be low in fat, which is not true of many of our most popular protein foods. The average hamburger patty, for example, is approximately 65 percent fat. The average hot dog is about 70 percent fat. Even a seemingly low-fat broiled chicken breast (including skin) is in the neighborhood of 40 percent fat. To be fat-burning, our proteins need to be put on a "diet."

"If a high-fat meal is followed by inactivity or, worse yet, going to bed, it takes fat cells only four to eight hours to absorb most of the fat that's been taken in."

Ronald M. Krauss, M.D., Chairman of the Nutrition Committee for the American Heart Association

This can be done with proper cooking techniques in some cases, trimming off skin and visible fat in others, or simply opting for low-fat versions of such foods as milk, yogurt, and cheese. We'll be looking more closely at how to buy and prepare fat-burning foods, but we offer now the following list to get you at least thinking in the right direction. These are high-protein foods that do not come in the company of lots of fat. Most are less than 20 percent fat and therefore within permissible (edible) limits.

Food	Percent of Calories from Fat
Egg whites (and most egg substitutes)	0
Yogurt, non-fat	3
Skim milk	5
Low-fat (one percent fat) cottage cheese	13
Low-fat fish and shellfish:	
Tuna (packed in water)	3
Cod	5
Haddock	5
Lobster	5
Scallops	8
Shrimp	10
Clams	12
Flounder	12
Snapper	12
Sole	12
Perch	16
Monkfish	18
Halibut	19
Trout	26
Turkey (light meat, no skin, roasted)	8
Chicken (white meat, no skin, broiled)	19
Pork (tenderloin, broiled)	26
Beef (top round, broiled)	28

Fiber: Different Types For Different Gripes

When you think of fiber, what comes to mind? The indigestible roughage in foods such as wheat bran that "passes right through you"?

Congratulations for being half right. That sort of fiber is known as "insoluble" fiber and it does, in fact, pass through the digestive tract essentially unchanged. This type of fiber fights constipation and hemorrhoids and reduces the risks of colon cancer by keeping the intestines clean of potentially cancer-causing compounds. This sweeping action also has been shown to help escort fats through the intestines before their calories have time to be fully absorbed, thus making insoluble fiber an invaluable addition to a weight-loss program.

But fiber comes in a "soluble" form, too, principally in fruits, vegetables, beans, and whole grains. Its area of impact is not so much the bowels as the blood. Studies show that soluble fiber can help lower cholesterol levels and keep levels of insulin stable. This helps control hunger and how readily calories can move into fat cells to be stored. Consequently, soluble fiber is as essential to weight loss as its insoluble cousin, but it's the two types working together that make a truly dynamic, fat-fighting duo.

Studies show that our current intake of fiber (of both types) averages approximately 10 to 15 grams a day, a far cry from the 25 to 30 grams nutritionists say we should be getting for overall health and weight control.

View the following list with 25 to 30 grams in mind and try gradually to include more of these foods in your diet. (For the beginner, high-fiber foods can cause flatulence and bloating, so go slow if these foods have yet to become a regular part of your diet.)

Food	Serving Size	Fiber (Grams)
Apple	1 medium	7.9
Barley (cooked)	$^1/_2$ cup	12.3
Blackberries	1 cup	7.2
Broccoli	medium stalk	7.4
Corn bran	2 tablespoons	7.9
Oat bran	2 tablespoons	3.0
Rice bran	2 tablespoons	2.3
Wheat bran	2 tablespoons	1.8
Chick peas	$^1/_2$ cup	7.0
Currants	$^1/_2$ cup	4.9
Figs, dried	3 figs	5.2
Kidney beans	$^1/_2$ cup	6.9
Lentils	$^1/_2$ cup	5.2
Lima beans	$^1/_2$ cup	6.8
Navy beans	$^1/_2$ cup	4.9
Peas	$^1/_2$ cup	4.2
Potato	1 medium	3.9
Raspberries	1 cup	6.0
Spinach	$^1/_2$ cup	5.7
Succotash	$^1/_2$ cup	5.2

(Note: Although not on the list due to slightly lesser levels, virtually all fruits, vegetables, beans, and whole-grain cereals, and breads are good fiber sources and should be part of a fat-fighting diet.)

Know Your Daily Fat "Budget"

The following chart can help you keep your fat intake in the healthful neighborhood of 25 percent of the calories you consume. Simply locate your desired weight in the column at the left and find the corresponding number of grams of fat in the column at the right. This is the amount of fat you should not exceed per day to achieve that desired weight.

Women		Men	
Desired Weight:	Daily Fat Limit (In Grams)	Desired Weight:	Daily Fat Limit (In Grams)
110	37	130	51
120	40	140	54
130	43	150	58
140	47	160	62
150	50	170	66
160	53	180	70
170	57	190	74
180	60	200	78

Butter vs. Margarine: Both Losers

Is there a pat answer to the butter vs. margarine debate?

Yes: It's best to avoid them both. According to experts, both serve up a monstrous 11 grams of fat in a single teaspoon, and both have other unhealthful effects, especially margarine. That might come as a surprise, given margarine's "healthier" reputation. However, researchers at the Harvard School of Public Health and at the George Washington University Medical Center recently have completed studies that should have you thinking twice about margarine in your refrigerator.

Butter is loaded with saturated fat (the kind that increases risks of heart disease by raising levels of LDL, the bad cholesterol). Margarine is full of "trans-fatty acids," which are created when vegetable oil has been "hydrogenated" to make it firm enough to spread. Trans-fatty acids also have been shown to elevate LDL levels.

The bad news doesn't stop there, however. In addition to raising bad (LDL) cholesterol, trans-fatty acids have been shown to lower good (HDL) cholesterol—the kind that can reduce heart disease risks. Saturated fat, by comparison, has been found in some studies actually to raise levels of LDL.

So sorry, "oleo" fans. By raising the bad cholesterol and lowering the good, the type of fat found in margarine wins the dubious distinction of being the most hazardous to be found, proving perhaps that it really isn't nice to fool Mother Nature after all.

If, however, your taste buds *demand* butter or margarine, butter appears to be the more healthful—or the least harmful—of the two. But because butter is a saturated fat, it should be used in very small amounts.

(Note: Hydrogenated fats are found in other products as well. Learn to avoid them in vegetable shortening and many commercially prepared baked goods such as cookies, cakes, pastries, and pies. Always check a food's label to be sure.)

The Tortoise vs. The Hare: The Case of Linda

They shook hands precisely at midnight on New Year's Eve. The contest was to last one year, with a prize of $50 to the winner for every pound marking the margin of victory. Linda at 5'5" weighed 165, while Barbara, one inch taller, tipped the scales at 172.

Barbara decided to blast off from the start like a rocket and get a lead she could hang onto until the finish. Linda planned to go slow and easy and lose just half a pound a week.

Two weeks into the contest, Barbara announced that she had lost "10 big ones" by restricting herself to a salad and one diet milkshake a day. Linda, whose typical lunch was a bowl of bean soup and homemade whole wheat bread, had lost just two pounds.

Because they worked for the same company, the two saw each other often. Barbara would poke her head into Linda's office each Monday morning and hold up her fingers to show the new total of her losses. But one Monday Barbara phoned in sick—"sick" as in totally demoralized. She had succumbed to a major "binge" over the weekend. The weight she so agonizingly had lost began to return almost visibly. Worse yet, she had lost so much muscle tissue during the course of her nearly four-month-long "fast," she had trouble losing any more weight despite limiting herself to 800 calories a day.

Linda, meanwhile, had stayed true to her half-pound-a-week plan, losing 8 pounds painlessly over the four months the contest had lasted.

Moral of the story: Patience may be your greatest weight-loss ally. Go slow if where you're going is a place you plan to stay.

The Calories in Cocktails:
Nothing to Celebrate

Where does alcohol fit into an effective weight-loss picture?

As more of a road block than many of us realize, says Dr. John P. Foreyt, of the Nutrition Research Clinic at the Baylor College of Medicine. Foreyt believes that drinking alcohol has essentially the same effect on body weight as does eating fat. "Alcohol may not show up as a layer of oil on top of a glass of water, but in terms of how it's metabolized, it's a lot more like fat than it is a carbohydrate."

Alcohol's calories alone argue this point: 7 calories per gram (fat has 9) as compared with 4 calories per gram for carbohydrates and protein. The higher a drink's alcohol content, the higher the calorie count, as the following chart shows:

Beverage	Portion	% of Alcohol	Calories by Volume
Beer (regular)	12 oz.	5	146
Beer (light)	12 oz.	4	99
Liquor (bourbon, gin, rum, scotch, vodka)	1.5 oz.	40	97
Wine (dry)	3.5 oz.	11.5	73
Wine (sweet fortified, such as port, sherry, and sweet vermouth)	3.5 oz.	18-19	140

Making alcohol's calories even more "fattening," moreover, is their lack of patience when it comes to being metabolized. When you eat an 800-calorie meal along with a couple of glasses of dry wine (about 150 calories), it's the calories in the wine that are first digested. What this does to the 800 calories in the meal is make them that much more available to be stored as fat rather than burned as energy.

Then, too, alcohol has a tendency to reduce inhibitions—including those responsible for portion control. Studies show that people are more likely to overeat when they've been "primed" with a couple of cocktails. Not surprisingly, they tend to overindulge in fatty foods especially.

"Pub Grub" Packs on the Pounds, Too

But it's not just the calories in our drinks that can give rise to a beer belly. The calories in those "can't have just one" bar snacks add to the swell, too.

	Calories	Grams of Fat	% of Calories from Fat
1 cup peanuts	1,146	72	76
5 buffalo wings	860	55	58
30 corn chips (about 1 oz.)	155	9	53
30 potato chips (about 2 oz.)	315	21	61

Better choices: Air-popped, unbuttered popcorn (12 percent fat) and pretzels (10 percent fat).

10 Commandments For Making Weight Loss Last

Today's leading nutritionists believe that the following are the ten most important strategies for losing weight, not just permanently but painlessly—without hunger, without cravings, and without weakness or fatigue.

1. **Avoid getting hungry.** That's right—no meal skipping allowed. That might sound like weight-loss heresy, but it's not. Your body will adjust its metabolic rate to burn fewer calories if you allow yourself to be chronically famished. You're also likely to overcompensate when you do eat, thinking you "deserve" it, and thus negate any benefit from your misery.

2. **Nibble, don't gorge.** Ever noticed how some people can snack constantly but can still maintain a desirable weight? It's not a mirage. It's been proven that eating small meals produces less of an insulin response from the pancreas. This is good news for the waistline because the job of insulin is to help calories get stored as fat.

3. **Limit, but do not eliminate, dietary fat.** Some fat is necessary to absorb fat-soluble vitamins, such as vitamins A, D, and E. Some fat also is needed to slow down the rate at which carbohydrates and proteins are metabolized, thus helping to stave off hunger. Notice that we said "some." All of the benefits of dietary fat could be achieved with levels as low as 10 percent of total calories,

but that's a level that most people would find severe. Dietary fat levels in the 20 to 30 percent range are more acceptable.

4. **Know your "good" carbohydrates from your "bad."** If all carbohydrates were nutritionally equal, a bowl of table sugar would be as healthful as a baked potato. But while sugar is a "simple" carbohydrate (meaning it digests quickly and has no significant nutrients or fiber), the potato is a "complex" carbohydrate that delivers a wide range of energizing nutrients the body digests more slowly.

5. **Learn to slim down your proteins.** Protein is critical to your fat-burning diet because it helps maintain muscle cells, which burn fat for energy. Equally important, protein helps block fat storage by keeping insulin levels low, and it provides feelings of fullness by preventing carbohydrates from being metabolized too quickly.

6. **Fill up on fiber.** Because fiber does not fully digest, it tends to be exceptionally filling, despite being very low in calories and virtually free of fat. Better yet, insoluble (cannot be dissolved) fiber acts like a janitor by grabbing onto fats in the intestines and sweeping them out of the body before they can be fully absorbed. Diets high in insoluble fiber can reduce caloric absorption by as much as 3 percent—enough, on a 2,000-calorie diet, to allow you 60 calories absolutely "free." Soluble (dissolvable) fiber, which quells hunger by stabilizing insulin levels in the blood, is no fat-fighting slouch either.

7. **Impound your bathroom scale.** The loss of true body fat, which is lighter in weight than either muscle tissue or water, might not be evident when you step on your scale. Some people even wind up weighing more when they lose body fat, especially if they exercise, because they gain muscle in place of the lost fat.

8. **Exercise, don't agonize.** Exercise is critical to long-term weight loss, as we'll be seeing in more detail in Chapter 3. But the only exercise that's going to work is the exercise you're going to do consistently. Engage in activities you enjoy and involve friends or family members whenever possible. Research shows that exercising within approximately 30 minutes of eating can boost calorie burning by as much as 10 percent.

9. **Don't let small slips become major slides.** Maybe you know the scenario all too well: One chocolate chip cookie becomes two, becomes three, becomes a bowl of ice cream. Suddenly, with weeks' worth of work down the drain, you figure you should pack in your weight-loss effort and try again another day. But don't panic. By sticking to a low-fat diet, you can afford such misdemeanors. In fact, one study found that people on low-fat diets experienced no ill effects despite eating "splurge" meals (a ham and cheese sandwich and a milkshake) as often as once every other day.

10. **Eat light at night.** Sorry, midnight snackers, but studies show that calories consumed shortly before bed will more than likely become fat because there simply isn't enough competition from your body's muscle cells when you're in dreamland to encourage them to do much else. Many weight-loss experts recommend putting a padlock on your appetite after about 7:00 PM. If you find that you need a before-bed snack to help you sleep, make it as low in fat as possible: a glass of skim milk, some nonfat or low-fat yogurt, a small bowl of cereal, or a piece of fresh fruit.

CHAPTER 2

TIPS FOR A LEANER LIFESTYLE

Of course there's more to permanent weight loss than just knowing the right foods to eat. First, you must actually eat the food—both consistently and enthusiastically. The more a diet asks you to deprive yourself, after all, the more likely it is to fail.

Then, too, there are the challenges of dealing with issues other than food. Less than supportive family members ("why can't we call for pizza?"). Or undeniable cravings for sweets. Or those times when life's stresses weigh on your weight-loss efforts with the force of a giant pound cake.

Relax. If you've got the will, we've got the way. In this chapter, you'll learn the "nuts and bolts" of what it takes to get a successful weight-control program going—and keep it going. The secret to sticking to any weight-loss program lies in being determined but also in being flexible—in learning to bend, not break. Just because you slip doesn't mean you have to fall.

So What Should You Weigh, Anyway?

The $64,000 question is: What is my ideal weight?

More and more, doctors are beginning to realize that it's not an easy question to answer. Until recently it was thought that our weight should be within the standards established by insurance companies based on what is average for most Americans. However, the fallacy of this approach now is being understood because it says nothing about why we weigh what we do. A football player who exercises strenuously and eats a healthful low-fat diet could be considered overweight purely by virtue of being heavily muscled. A "couch potato" who is primarily bones and flab, on the other hand, could be considered at a healthy weight despite having a terrible diet and getting no exercise at all.

FAT-BURNING FACT:

Four out of ten adults currently weigh at least 20 percent more than they should. This computes to be 2.5 billion pounds of excess body fat— the weight of approximately 300,000 adult hippos.

Nor do the "ideal" weight charts say anything about where our extra pounds are located, which research is now showing to be very important. People who tend to carry their extra weight in their abdomens appear to be at greater risks for heart disease, diabetes, and certain forms of cancer than people who carry their surplus poundage on their hips, buttocks, and thighs. It's riskier to be shaped like an apple, in other words, than a pear.

But why should people shaped like apples be at a greater health risk than people shaped like pears?

The reason has to do with the difference in the metabolic activity of what doctors have recently identified as two distinctly different types of fat. People with large, apple-shaped midsections usually have a high percentage of what is known as "visceral" fat—fat located inside, as opposed to outside, the abdominal wall. Because this type of fat is close to vital organs such as the liver, gallbladder, and pancreas, it's thought to influence risks of diabetes and heart disease by adversely affecting levels of fat, cholesterol, and insulin in the blood.

This is not the case, however, with the other more visible type of fat called "subcutaneous" fat, which lies underneath the skin but outside the abdominal wall. Because it is not as close to vital organs as visceral fat, subcutaneous fat appears not to have similar health risks. This is ironic given that subcutaneous fat is the type we most despise because of its greater visibility. People with this type of fat usually are pear-shaped.

Are both types of fat equal in terms of the efforts needed to lose them?

Thankfully, no. Because of its greater metabolic involvement, visceral fat appears to be more responsive than subcutaneous fat to diet and exercise. When you begin following the recommendations given in this book, therefore, you may take comfort in knowing that you'll be burning fat where it counts most. Yes, the unwanted fat on your hips and thighs also will be diminished, but your most dangerous, internal, fat will be the first to feel the brunt of your efforts.

Your Best "Fighting" Weight: One You Don't Have to Fight

This brings us to an important point that you should keep in mind as you begin to incorporate fat-burning strategies into your life. By eating a nutritious low-fat diet and getting at least 30 minutes of physical activity each day, you'll achieve a weight that is "ideal" because it will be the weight best suited for helping you achieve ideal health. If the figure you achieve is not the one of your dreams, blame your genes. Some of us are simply born to carry more body fat than others, and new research shows this does not necessarily have to be unhealthful.

What does matter are the lifestyle factors responsible for our weights. Someone who keeps his or her weight down by skipping meals, taking diet pills, or smoking is going to be less healthy than someone who may be plump despite eating well and being physically active. As Dr. Steven Blair of the Cooper Institute of Aerobics Research said, "Healthy bodies come in all shapes and sizes. We need to stop hounding people about their weight and encourage them to eat well and exercise."

How Healthful Is Your Diet?
Take This Test and Find Out

Before we go further, we need to know what your current eating habits are. If you're like most Americans, they probably need some work. While we've begun to make some progress in our efforts to cut down on fat—by reducing our average food intake from 38 percent of calories from fat down to 34—we still have a way to go to reach the level of 25 percent that most nutritionists now recommend. Considering that we've actually gotten heavier in recent years despite making this cutback, it's clear that we may need to reduce our calorie intake overall. Take the following test and see how you fare.

1. **My usual pattern of eating is to:**
   a. eat a healthful breakfast, ample lunch, and a small dinner interspersed with healthful snacks in between
   b. sit down to three fairly traditional "square" meals a day
   c. skip breakfast or lunch and have a big dinner
   d. skip breakfast *and* lunch and have a huge dinner

2. **In an average day I will have the following number of servings of vegetables:**
   a. four or more
   b. two or three
   c. one
   d. I despise vegetables and eat them rarely, if ever

3. **In an average day I will have the following number of servings or pieces of fresh fruit:**
   a. four or more
   b. two or three
   c. one
   d. usually none

4. **The type of bread I usually eat is:**
   a. whole-grain bread that I make myself with no added fat
   b. whole-grain bread I buy at a bakery
   c. whole wheat, pumpernickel, or rye from the supermarket
   d. white bread from the supermarket

5. **The breakfast that most closely resembles my usual one is:**
   a. a high-fiber, vitamin-fortified cereal with skim milk and a piece of fresh fruit
   b. frozen waffles with butter and syrup and a glass of juice
   c. eggs with bacon or sausage and buttered toast
   d. a piece of pastry and coffee or no breakfast at all

6. **The way I most often eat potatoes is:**
   a. baked, with yogurt or a tiny bit of butter as a topping
   b. mashed, with butter and/or a gravy topping
   c. French-fried, with ketchup
   d. French-fried, with a melted cheese topping

7. **Most of the protein in my diet comes from:**
   a. chicken or turkey (skinless) and/or fish, usually baked or broiled
   b. beef and pork
   c. cheese and other full-fat dairy products
   d. fast-food entrees such as hamburgers and hot dogs

8. **The milk I usually drink or use on my cereal is:**
   a. skim
   b. 1% fat
   c. 2% fat
   d. regular

9. **When pan-frying, I'll use:**
   a. a non-stick pan so that I won't need to use any fat at all
   b. a little bit of olive or vegetable oil
   c. a little bit of butter
   d. a lot of butter or lard

10. **The amount of water I drink in an average day is:**
    a. six eight-ounce glasses, or more
    b. four to six eight-ounce glasses
    c. two to four eight-ounce glasses
    d. fewer than two glasses

11. **The number of times in an average week I eat at a fast-food restaurant is:**
    a. I avoid eating at fast-food restaurants
    b. one
    c. two or three
    d. four or more

12. **My favorite between-meal or TV-time snacks are:**
    a. fresh vegetable crudités and/or fresh fruit
    b. saltless pretzels, rice cakes, or popcorn
    c. potato or corn chips
    d. cookies, pastry, or candy

13. **The number of cans or bottles of non-diet soda I'll have in an average day is:**
    a. zero
    b. one or two
    c. three or four
    d. more than four

14. **I give into the urge to have a really decadent dessert:**
    a. rarely
    b. about once a month
    c. about once a week
    d. I am having a really decadent dessert right now

SCORING:

Give yourself a one for every "a" answer, a two for every "b," a three for every "c," and a four for every "d."

15–22: High Honors. Congratulations! Your diet is truly a fat-burning marvel that is giving your body every health advantage it deserves.

23–30: Honors. Good work. Your diet is to be commended, although there still are improvements you could make.

31–38: Honorable Mention. Your diet is fair, but nothing special. You could be leaner, healthier, and enjoy more energy by making the changes suggested in this book.

39–46: Less Than Honorable Mention. Careful. Your diet borders on the risky and could affect your health adversely. You owe it to yourself to make the changes suggested in this book.

47 and above: Dishonorable Mention. Shame on you. Your diet is a disgrace and is definitely bad for your health. You had better hurry up and change your eating habits.

FAT-BURNING FACT:

A small, steady supply of food during the day keeps insulin levels steadier, so that your brain doesn't turn up your appetite and send signals to fat cells to store more fat.

In The Bag:

Best Strategies for Fighting Fat in the Supermarket

Now that you have a pretty good picture of your present eating habits, it's time to do something about them.

Let's start where every weight-loss effort should start—at the supermarket. You can't eat what you haven't bought. By buying the right food, you can avoid those showdowns with your willpower that occur when you're tired and stressed and that cheesecake in your refrigerator looks awfully good. Shop smart and you will prevent the "enemy" from entering your home and tempting you. Following are some strategies to help you do precisely that:

Do not shop when you're hungry. Shopping on an empty stomach can lead to a heaping shopping cart faster than you can say, "But the sticky buns were on sale!" Try to shop as close after eating a satisfying meal as possible. That way, your brain will dictate your purchases, not your stomach.

Always shop with a list. This, too, can discourage unwise food choices spurred by impulse buying. Compile your list when you're feeling comfortable and have time to concentrate on the consequences of what you'll be buying. Do you really need that half gallon of mint chocolate chip ice cream? Better to be safe than sorry.

Try not to shop with your children. Nothing against the little ones, but they can "fatten" up a shopping cart in the blink of an eye. Get a babysitter if you have to; the cost will be covered by the cupcakes and marshmallow cereal you won't be pressured to buy.

61

Do not be swayed by food coupons or by special money-saving bargains. It certainly can be tempting to put thriftiness ahead of health, but is anything really a bargain if it's bad for you? Think about that the next time the bags of potato chips or chocolate donuts are two-for-one. Your goal should be maximum nutrition for your food dollar, not just calories.

Buy fresh or frozen foods rather than canned. This applies to meats and fish as well as vegetables and fruits. Not only will you get better taste and in many cases superior nutrition, you'll get less sodium. This is a plus for the estimated 20 percent of the population for whom too much salt can result in high blood pressure.

Buy in quantity if you're also getting quality. If you come across a special on particularly healthful foods—low-fat meats, fish, poultry, fruits, or vegetables (fresh or frozen)—stock up, by all means. Not only will you be saving money, you'll be assuring that these healthful foods eventually will end up on your table.

Know your best low-fat bargains. Have you ever noticed how little a 10-pound bag of potatoes costs—or dried beans, rice, or pasta? These are fantastic food bargains. Your low-fat diet also can be a low-cost diet, so don't pass these foods by.

Avoid the "enemy." Just as there are foods tailor-made to burn fat, there also are those that will very easily become fat. The best way to avoid being tempted by the latter is not to allow them into your home in the first place. Foremost among these foods are butter, shortening, margarine, regular mayonnaise, hard cheeses, whole milk, sour cream, salad dressings (except for low and non-fat), ice cream, bacon, sausage, luncheon meats (except for sliced turkey or chicken breast), creamy soups, corn and potato chips, and high-fat cuts of beef, poultry, and pork. (See next page.)

Learn the fine art of substitution. Acting in response to the concerns of today's health-conscious consumers, the food industry has come up with non-fat or low-fat versions of everything from soup to nuts. Add to these the low-fat foods offered by Mother Nature, and it quickly becomes clear that your supermarket offers a tremendous variety to choose from when putting together low-fat meals.

FAT-BURNING FACT:

Research shows that by reducing the fat in their diets, most people can lower their blood cholesterol levels by 10 to 15 percent—enough to reduce their risks of heart disease by 20 to 30 percent!

The following are healthful substitutes for unhealthful staples:

Head right for:	Pass on by:	Grams of fat saved per serving
Air-popped popcorn (12%)*	Potato chips (61%)	6.8
Beef, top round roast (26%)	Ground chuck (66%)	16.0
Canned tuna, in water (3%)	Canned tuna, in oil (45%)	5.5
Fresh flounder (12%)	Flounder filets, breaded and fried (49%)	26.0
Fresh fruit (2–10%)	Cookies, chocolate chip (40%)	10.5
Low-fat cheese (36%)	Regular cheese (77%)	7.0
Low-fat mayonnaise (40%)	Regular mayonnaise (98%)	10.0
Non-fat egg substitute (0%)	Eggs (61%)	5.0
Non-fat frozen yogurt (0%)	Ice cream (54%)	11.5
Non-fat yogurt (3%)	Regular yogurt (48%)	7.0
Pork tenderloin (26%)	Pork chops (51%)	7.6
Skim milk (6%)	Whole milk (49%)	8.3
Skinless chicken breasts (19%)	Chicken legs (40%)	5.0
Sliced turkey breast (13%)	Sliced ham (52%)	5.3

*Percentage indicates fat content.

Best and Worst Picks

Beef

Best	Worst
Top Round (29% fat)	Ribs (75% fat)
Eye of Round (30% fat)	Chuck Blade Roast (72% fat)
Top Sirloin (36% fat)	T-Bone Steak (68% fat)
Filet Mignon (38% fat)	Porterhouse Steak (64% fat)

Pork

Best	Worst
Center Loin Pork Chops (26% fat)	Loin Blade Steaks (50% fat)
Tenderloin (26% fat)	Ribs (54% fat)
	Shoulder Blade Steaks (51% fat)

Poultry

Best	Worst
Turkey—light meat (19% fat without skin; 38% with skin)	Turkey—dark meat (35% fat without skin; 47% fat with skin)
Chicken—light meat (23% fat without skin; 44% with skin)	Chicken—dark meat (43% fat without skin; 56% fat with skin)

Slim Cookin's

Once nutritional low-fat food has been purchased, we must make sure it stays that way. What happens to that food in your kitchen can make or break low-fat fare. How healthful, after all, is a 12-percent-fat flounder filet if it's been breaded, deep-fried, and smothered in tartar sauce?

At about 50 percent fat—even without the 98-percent-fat tartar sauce!—not very. Even the foods that are most healthful can become little better than "junk" food if the preparation is too "heavy-handed."

That said, the following are the best methods for keeping your cooking "lite:"

Best fat-fighting cooking techniques

ⓒ *Broiling.* Broiling is a good fat-fighter—especially if done on a rack or in a pan that allows fat to drain away from what's being cooked.

ⓒ *Baking.* Also a good fat-fighter, but, as with broiling, it's best done in a pan with a slightly raised rack to allow the fat to drain.

ⓒ *Poaching.* Another good low-fat technique (especially for fish) because fat has a tendency to leach into the poaching liquid.

ⓒ *Grilling* (outdoor barbecues included). A fat-fighter extraordinaire, as fat drains into and helps fuel the very fire doing the cooking!

⏲ *Steaming.* Your best fat-free way to cook vegetables.

⏲ *Microwaving.* A very good fat-free way to cook practically anything.

Note: The cooking methods you should avoid are pan-frying, deep-frying, and braising or sautéing in butter or oil.

Best fat-fighting "weapons"

To employ the best fat-fighting cooking techniques, it can help immensely to have your kitchen "armed" with the right fat-fighting equipment. Following are the utensils that can best serve you:

- non-stick frying pans and bake ware

- a ridged grill pan for cooking burgers, chops, and fish

- steaming baskets for steaming vegetables

- a fat-skimmer for skimming the surface fat from soups and gravies

- a fat-free (hot-air style) popcorn popper

- a blender (for making low-fat soups, sauces, and shakes)

- a set of good knives (for chopping fresh vegetables and trimming all visible fat from meats)

- a microwave oven (a great low-fat cooking method)

- plastic storage bags (for freezing low-fat foods purchased in bulk)

- a good collection of low-fat cookbooks

Mealtime Tips for a Trimmer You

Even the most healthful foods can lead to weight gain if we grossly overindulge. So it's important to practice a certain restraint at mealtime. This does not mean depriving yourself, but it does mean learning how to stop eating when you've had your biological fill, something many overeaters fail to do. Here are some helpful strategies if a runaway appetite sometimes poses a problem for you:

Eat slowly. Studies show that it takes approximately 20 minutes for your stomach to tell your brain it's full, so pace your eating accordingly. Take small rather than large bites and chew each bite thoroughly before swallowing. What you want to avoid is the "I can't believe I ate the whole thing" syndrome that happens when you eat too quickly.

Serve meals piping hot. Not only will this slow down the rate at which you eat, hot foods tend to be more satisfying because the heat accentuates their flavors.

Pay attention when you eat. Eating while doing other things, such as watching TV or reading, can have you stuffed in no time. Arrange to have your meals in a calm, relaxing atmosphere and concentrate totally on what you're eating.

Take breaks to breathe. By stopping periodically during a meal to take five or so deep breaths, you'll not only interrupt the mindless "cruise control" approach to dining, you'll help arrest your hunger because your expanding diaphragm will help you get a better "feel" for the amount of food you've actually put into your stomach.

Put leftovers away quickly. The longer leftovers linger, the more likely you'll be to pick at them, so the sooner you can get them out of sight and into your refrigerator, the better.

Drink lots of water with your meals. It's a great way to fill up and 100 percent fat- and calorie-free.

"Eat" lots of water with your meals. We're talking about low-calorie vegetables and salads—great ways to munch and crunch without a lot of caloric dues to pay.

Don't desert dessert. Satisfy post-meal sweet cravings with a low-fat sherbet, low-fat frozen yogurt, Jell-O, or a serving of fresh fruit.

Pay attention to portions. Research has demonstrated that most people underestimate the amount of food they eat in a day, primarily because they have no clear understanding of how large a "serving" actually is. To assist you in this regard, we suggest that you think of servings in the following, visual terms:

- One serving of meat or fish usually constitutes two to three ounces, a portion roughly the size of a deck of cards.

- One serving of cheese usually refers to about $1^1/2$ ounces, a piece approximately the size of three dominoes.

- One serving of pasta, rice, vegetables, or mashed potatoes usually constitutes $1/2$ a cup, a portion about the size of half a baseball.

Eating Light When Eating Out

But will following a fat-burning diet mean you'll have to curb your appetite when eating out—especially at your favorite fast-food restaurant?

The answer to that depends on you. If you insist on having it truly "your way" when you eat out, restaurant dining needn't be a problem. However, you will need to be knowledgeable and assertive about which dishes you should avoid.

The following are some fat-fighting strategies worth remembering, whether you're eating beneath the Golden Arches or at a four-star restaurant in Paris.

- *Try to avoid smorgasbords or all-you-can-eat buffets.* Not only do these formats encourage you to overeat, they allow you little opportunity to request changes in the way the food is prepared.

- *Order a la carte.* You benefit from greater variety this way, and you avoid the temptation to overeat when served a meal that is larger than you might like.

- *Call ahead.* This is especially advisable if you're not sure about the healthfulness of the food a restaurant serves or about its willingness to make changes.

- *Don't be afraid to be assertive.* It can be easy to worry about sounding "picky" when you request changes to a menu, but one simple fact can help make you bold: Most restaurants want your business and usually will do anything reasonably possible to get it.

⊙ *Don't be afraid to be inquisitive.* A cheeseburger is easy, but when dishes become more complex and are given names in a foreign language, confusion can reign. This needn't be a problem if you're willing to ask your waitress or waiter what ingredients go into the dish and how it's prepared. If all you get is shrugged shoulders, don't be afraid to ask if you can talk with the chef.

⊙ *Be wary of appetizers.* They can seem like a good idea as "just a little something to tide you over," but many are high in fat as well as brimming with enough calories to qualify as an entree. If you do need to nibble on something, stick to bread or order a cup of low-fat soup.

⊙ *Order sauces and salad dressings on the side.* Whether it's gravy for your roast beef, Hollandaise sauce for your broccoli, or blue cheese dressing for your salad, you'll have a lot more control if *you* decide the amount.

⊙ *Know your friendly from your "fiendish" pastas.* Pasta in a tomato sauce is one thing, but pasta smothered in a creamy cheese sauce is another story entirely. If you have questions about a pasta sauce, be sure to ask how it's made.

⊙ *Forego rich desserts.* Unless a fresh-fruit dish or sherbet is being offered, you could be looking at more fat and calories than were in your entree.

Food Labels In Focus

Learn how to read—and understand—nutritional labels. Nearly all foods now have them, and they're a dream come true for the health-conscious and the weight-conscious alike. Following are the most important things to look for:

The amount of fat a serving contains. This will be presented to you in two ways: the number of grams of fat the food has and the number of calories that fat contains. (If this latter figure computes* to be more than about 25 percent of the food's total calories, consider it a high-fat food that you either should not buy or should eat in moderation only.)

The amount of fiber the food contains. This will be listed in grams and also as "% of daily value." Because you should be getting between 25 and 35 grams of fiber in your diet daily, any food with a fiber content of approximately three grams or more per serving (or 10% of your daily value) should be deemed a wise fiber choice.

The percentages of vitamins and minerals the food contains. These will be listed toward the end of the label and, as with the food's other nutrients, will reflect the degree to which the food satisfies your daily needs as expressed by "% of daily value."(If a vitamin or mineral is not listed, it will be because the food's "daily value" is less than two percent.)

To make this calculation, divide the food's total number of calories per serving by the number of its calories that come from fat. As mentioned, any food that turns out to be approximately 25 percent fat or above should be excluded from your diet or eaten sparingly.

FAT-BURNING FACT:

Skim milk gets 5 percent of its calories from fat, while whole milk gets 51 percent from fat. More than 30 percent calories from fat increases risks of heart disease, obesity, and cancer.

Taking the Fat out of Fast Food

If you're like most American families, 40 percent of your food budget gets spent on eating out, and a whopping portion of that goes toward the burgers and fries. Should you avoid fast-food restaurants?

That depends on what you order and how much. While many of the items offered at these eateries could blow your entire daily fat budget in just one serving—a Double Whopper with cheese from Burger King, for example, serves up a mammoth 55 grams of fat in addition to nearly 900 calories—other fast-food entrees are actually quite lean. Wendy's grilled chicken sandwich, for example, has only 7 grams of fat and a modest 290 calories.

It helps to know what you're biting into at fast-food restaurants. The following fast-food eating tips and the nutritional chart should help you make fast food, fit food.

Think small. Avoid entrees labeled "jumbo," "giant," or "deluxe." As these adjectives imply, the number of calories and grams of fat in these monstrosities are astronomical.

Think plain. The sauce on the featured sandwich may be "gourmet," but it's not without a price. These sauces are largely mayonnaise, which is nearly 100 percent fat. If it's a burger you want, have it plain or piled with fat-free lettuce and tomato.

Fear the deep-fryer. The chicken or fish sandwich might seem to be a healthier choice than a burger, but not if it's been in the fryer first. Burger King's broiled chicken sandwich has only 10 grams of fat and 280 calories, for example, while its deep-fried fish cousin has 32 grams of fat and 620 calories.

When ordering chicken, think of "extra crispy" as extra crumbly. It's hard to believe, but the crispier the coating, the higher its fat content. If you want chicken and fried is the only way it's offered, put manners aside and remove the coating before eating. Your heart as well as your waistline will thank you.

Chase down the chili. Most chili dishes at fast-food restaurants are less than 30 percent fat and loaded with heart-healthy fiber, thanks to the beans.

Know your friends from your enemies at the salad bar. All those greens and vegetables are great, but don't make the mistake of sabotaging them with salad dressings that easily add as many as 200 calories per tablespoon. Use vinegar or low-calorie dressings instead. Try to avoid the mayonnaise-based potato salads and coleslaws; choose instead vinegar-based red beets, three-bean salad, or chow-chow. Other healthful, low-fat choices include bean sprouts, chick peas, cottage cheese, and hard-boiled eggs (providing you can avoid the yolk).

Pick low-fat toppings for your pizza. While a single slice of regular pizza without any trimmings has only about 10 grams of fat, piling on the pepperoni and extra cheese can double that. If it's toppings you must have, choose veggies such as mushrooms, green peppers, and onions.

Visit at mealtimes only. With the average fast-food meal coming in at 685 calories, it's important to consider it just that: a meal, not a snack. But if you do go a bit overboard, don't panic. Just be all the more careful about the fat and calories you consume in your other meals that day.

Fast Food Entrees:
The Good, The Bad, and the Abominable

The above are some general guidelines for having both your good health and your fast food. Now for some specifics. Here's a quick rundown of entrees containing ten or fewer grams of fat per serving. Any entree not on this list is too high in fat to be recommended as part of a fat-burning diet.

Arby's	Light Roast Chicken Deluxe
	Light Roast Turkey Deluxe
	Light Roast Beef Deluxe
	Roast Chicken Salad
Burger King	Broiler Chicken Sandwich
	Hamburger (small)
Dairy Queen	Beef Barbecue Sandwich
	Grilled Chicken Filet Sandwich
Domino's	Pizza (plain)
Hardee's	Real West Beef Barbecue Sandwich
	Grilled Chicken Breast Sandwich
	Turkey Sub
	Roast Beef Sub
	Ham Sub
	Combo Sub
Jack-in-the-Box	Chicken Fajita Pita
Long John Silver's	Baked Fish With Lemon Crumb
	Chicken Light Herb
	Gumbo with Cod
	Seafood Chowder

McDonald's	Hamburger (small)
	McLean Deluxe
	Chicken Fajitas
Pizza Hut	Thin 'N Crispy Pizza (plain)
	Veggie Lovers Pizza
Subway	Turkey Breast Sub
	Ham and Cheese Sub
	Veggie and Cheese Sub
Taco Bell	Chicken Taco (soft)
	Chicken Fajita
Wendy's	Grilled Chicken Sandwich
	Hamburger (junior)
	Chili

A word about those "sides." It's hard to believe but it's true: Most French fries served at fast-food restaurants are higher in fat than the hamburgers they accompany. The same is true of those seemingly innocent onion rings. At Burger King, for example, a small burger serves up 10 grams of fat and 260 calories while a medium serving of fries is good for 20 grams of fat and 372 calories. An order of Burger King onion rings: 19 grams of fat and 339 calories.

Olé! Eating Lean When Eating Ethnic

Do you enjoy "stretching" your palate by trying various ethnic dishes from time to time?

Good. Variety is the spice of a good diet, as well as of life. To keep your ethnic excursions as healthful as possible, however, it can help to know something about the items being offered. While some ethnic dishes can be very low in fat, others can be nutritional disasters. Here's a quick guide to help you separate the former from the latter.

Chinese: Many Chinese dishes are low in fat thanks to the predominance of rice and vegetables. Do be wary, however, of appetizers such as egg rolls, which usually are deep-fried. Stir-fried dishes generally are a good, low-fat choice—especially if you ask your chef to go easy on the oil. "Moo goo gai pan"—a combination of stir-fried mushrooms, bamboo shoots, water chestnuts, and chicken or seafood served over rice—is a particularly good choice. To be avoided: Peking duck with 30 grams of fat in just one $3^1/2$ ounce serving.

Mexican: Mexican fare also can be healthful and low in fat providing you avoid dishes smothered in cheese or sour cream. Also to be avoided is guacamole (made from high-fat avocados), refried beans (usually made with coconut oil or lard), and any entree that has been deep-fried or features beef or pork. Set your sights instead on vegetable and bean burritos, fresh-fish dishes, salsas, salads, unfried corn tortillas, beans, and rice.

Italian: Italian food is a case of Dr. Jekyll and Mr. Hyde: Many great low-fat dishes are available (any pasta dish served with a tomato-based marinara sauce, for example), but so are high-fat fiascoes such as "fettucini alfredo," made with cheese, heavy cream, and butter. Other good low-fat choices are vegetarian lasagna (providing you scrape off some of its surface cheese), "pollo cacciatore" (a boneless chicken breast served with a tomato and mushroom sauce), and "shrimp al vino blanco" (shrimp cooked in white wine). As for pizza, it can be as healthful as its toppings. Avoid extra cheese, pepperoni, and olives, opting instead for low-fat vegetables such as mushrooms, green peppers, and onions. High-protein foods like chicken, turkey, and shrimp also are fare game.

Indian: Like Italian food, Indian dishes also have their villains and heroes. Try to avoid dishes made with coconut oil or "ghee," a clarified butter. Look instead for entrees featuring ample amounts of beans, rice, onions, tomatoes, and bell peppers. One especially healthful dish is "murg jalfraize," made with plenty of spices, fresh vegetables, and skinless chicken.

"Haute" But Healthful: Low-Fat Fine Dining

Step up in the dining world, unfortunately, and you've often entered high-fat country. The reason is that costlier cuisines often borrow their cooking techniques from the French, who have never been stingy with butter and heavy cream. By learning the vocabulary associated with French cooking, however, you can avoid the most fat-filled offerings. Here's a list of terms you're most likely to encounter when choosing from a "four-star" menu:

The Vocabulary of Haute Cuisine

"ail"	garlic
"au gratin"	with cheese and bread crumbs
"beurre"	butter
"boeuf"	beef
"canard"	duck
"caneton"	duckling
"champignons"	mushrooms
"creme"	cream
"farci"	stuffed
"frit"	fried
"gigot"	lamb
"gratine"	baked with bread crumbs
"grille"	broiled
"jambon"	ham
"legumes"	vegetables
"mousse"	thickened with cream
"nouilles"	noodles
"oeufs"	eggs
"pané"	breaded

"poché"	poached
"pommes de terre"	potatoes
"porc"	pork
"poulet"	chicken
"quiche"	anything in a pie crust
"riz"	rice
"sauté"	cooked in small amount of oil quickly
"souffle"	with egg whites added
"veau"	veal
"vin"	wine

The most healthful entrees at French-based restaurants are seafood or poultry dishes that have been poached, baked, or broiled. If a sauce is offered, ask that it be served on the side.

FAT-BURNING FACT:

To reduce the fat and cholesterol you get from eggs, replace one whole egg in any type of cooking with two egg whites or the recommended portion of a commercial egg substitute.

Dining Low-Fat with the Family

There is more to eating healthfully than what goes into your own tummy, of course. If you have a family, you've got their dietary preferences to worry about. How do you prepare a dinner of low-fat poached fish for yourself when everybody else is clamoring for meatloaf and macaroni and cheese? Here are some ideas from nutritional experts.

○ *Have a family pow-wow.* It's important that you make clear to your family the importance of your dietary efforts, says Laurie Meyer, R.D., a spokesperson for the American Dietetic Association. Explain why you're making those efforts and suggest ways they can help. If they want nothing to do with your attempts at reform, warn them that they may have to do more cooking for themselves.

○ *Try winning them over gradually.* A "cook-for-yourself" policy would not work for young children, of course, so your approach to them—and to an apprehensive spouse—might be to compromise. So go ahead and make the meatloaf, but use ground turkey instead of beef. And make that macaroni dish but use low-fat cheese. Also, try other especially tasty low-fat meals, such as spaghetti in marinara sauce or herb-baked chicken, to help convert your family to a healthful way of eating. By proving that low-fat foods can be satisfyingly delicious, you could have them "on your side" before you know it.

◌ *Consider "yours" and "theirs."* If family members are not willing to compromise, then you may need to get tough, Meyer says. Tell your spouse he has to do his own cooking, as well as shopping, and inform your children that they either lean your way or settle for prepackaged convenience meals. A steady diet of canned ravioli can speak louder than words.

◌ *Give your family the same "pep talk" you give yourself.* Explain all the advantages of a low-fat diet—for reasons of health and weight control, for example—and follow up by asking for rational objections. If taste is all they can come up with, counter by whipping up a delicious low-fat version of a family favorite.

FAT-BURNING FACT:

The amount of refined sugar consumed by the average American adult in a single day: 20 teaspoons.

If You Can't Beat Them, Involve Them: The Case of Susan

Susan felt like she was fighting two battles. Not only was she having her own difficulties sticking to a low-fat diet, the resistance she was getting from her two hot-dog-and-hamburger-loving children, ages 7 and 10, was doubling her trouble.

So she decided to try a little "game." She invited her kids to help make a Chocolate-Banana Thick Shake (see recipe, p. 183). She then told them they could have a shake for dessert providing they peacefully ate whatever she served as the main course. To sweeten the deal even more, she invited her children to assist in the preparation of the main course whenever possible.

"I didn't have them wielding any sharp knives, that's for sure, but I did let them get involved with things like washing vegetables, stirring batters, and hand-forming tuna and turkey burgers," she says.

How'd it work out? "Actually a lot better than I expected," Susan says. "Granted, it meant more work for me—I had to come up with different low-fat desserts!—but it's been worth it because it's given us a chance to interact in ways we didn't before. We talk about school and their friends. We even talk about the importance of nutrition, which I've actually gotten them pretty interested in. They now picture fat as these greasy little creatures that like to hide in the blood vessels and join together to form dams to stop the flow of blood. My husband overheard us one night, and in all honesty I don't think he's had the same passion for fried foods since."

It's Not Just What You Eat, But How You Eat

Whether you're eating at home, at your local diner, or at a restaurant with linen tablecloths, cutting fat from your diet should be the primary goal of your weight-control efforts. But in addition to watching what you eat, you should be careful how you eat— and not just to avoid unwanted pounds. Studies show that eating "mini" meals frequently throughout the day—as many as six a day—can produce some decidedly "maxi" health benefits.

"Mini meals could well be one of the easiest and most effective healthy lifestyle changes that people can make," says Murray Mittleman, the director of the Institute for the Prevention of Cardiovascular Disease at Deaconess Hospital in Boston.

Dr. Mittleman points to research showing that eating small meals encourages the following important health benefits:

Weight control. As the size of a meal goes up, so does the proportion of calories stored as fat—the result of an overproduction of the fat-storing hormone called insulin. Infrequent eating also tends to produce overeating, as hunger often becomes hard to control. (One study of overweight people found that fully 80 percent were taking in fewer calories than people of normal weight, but they were making the "one-big-meal-a-day" mistake.)

Lower cholesterol. Eating small meals seems to create a more favorable environment for the digestion of dietary fats, cholesterol included. One experiment found that eating six small meals a day resulted in cholesterol reductions of 8 percent, which is enough to reduce risks of heart disease by 16 percent, according to David Jenkins, M.D., director of Clinical Nutrition and Risk Factor Modification at St. Michael's Hospital in Toronto.

Reduced risks of heart attacks and strokes. It's not imaginary that hospital emergency rooms experience a marked increase in the number of heart attacks on "feast" days such as Christmas and Thanksgiving. By demanding huge increases in the circulation of blood to the stomach, "very large meals can put the heart through a kind of digestive stress test," says Dr. Mittleman. In one study, a 280-calorie meal required an average of 21 gallons of blood from the hearts of test subjects, while a 720-calorie meal demanded 86 gallons—a difference large enough to fill the gas tank of the average car five times over! Large meals, and especially fatty ones, also can heighten the risks of heart attacks (and strokes) by increasing the danger of artery-clogging clots in the blood.

Prevention of heartburn. The smaller a meal, the less likely it is to "overflow" back into the esophagus—good news for heartburn sufferers. Eating smaller meals is the standard medical advice for victims of this condition, says Dr. Mittleman.

Greater energy and mental alertness. Small meals keep your body and brain supplied steadily with energy-producing glucose. This is not the case with large meals, which can produce drowsiness by drawing inordinate amounts of blood to the stomach, or skipping meals, which allows glucose (blood sugar levels) to drop too low.

Mastering the "Mini Meal"

Wait a minute. Six meals a day? If you're like most dieters, you probably think the best way to lose weight is to skip meals entirely. Get yourself good and hungry and your body will have no choice but to burn fat, right?

FAT-BURNING FACT:

The amount of body fat carried by the average American male is the caloric equivalent of 1,650 pancakes.

Wrong. As we have seen in Chapter 1, our bodies respond to hunger by attempting to preserve fat, not burn it. Avoiding hunger by eating mini meals, therefore, is actually far superior to starvation as a fat-burning strategy. It gives your body the energy it needs to burn fat the right way, which is through an active metabolism and an increase in physical activity.

Remember, too, that eating three meals a day is a relatively recent custom considering the estimated 50,000-year history of our species. For thousands of years we ate when we were hungry and not according to any predetermined plan. Some nutritionists argue that the convention of "three squares" is one of the reasons we've become so "round."

Fine, you say, but isn't it still a three-meal-a-day world?

Probably, but it doesn't have to be. Here are some tips for breaking free of the "three squares" pattern:

☺ *Divide before you devour.* The simplest way to turn three meals into six is to divide your breakfast, lunch, and dinner into two meals each. For breakfast, for example, have cereal with skim or low-fat milk, while saving a bagel and piece of fresh fruit for a mid-morning snack. For lunch, have your sandwich while reserving a cup of soup or a serving of low-fat yogurt for an afternoon treat. Dinner? Have your usual low-fat entree and side dishes, while saving your low-fat dessert for a snack an hour or so before bed.

☺ *Stock up on healthy snacks to eat at work.* Don't rely on the company vending machine. If you work at a desk, use it to store low-fat snacks such as individually packaged breakfast cereals, fresh or dried fruits, rice cakes, bagels, or slices of whole-grain bread. If your lunchroom has a refrigerator, use it to keep fresh vegetables, fruit juices, and containers of low-fat yogurt or cottage cheese. If you have access to a microwave, fire it up to make low-fat popcorn or instant soups.

☺ *Order appetizers rather than entrees when eating out.* This is an especially good idea if the entrees being offered could feed King Kong. Don't be afraid to order a more manageable appetizer and perhaps a salad or soup instead.

☺ *Pack healthful snacks for the road.* Why stop for over-priced junk food when you can pack healthful sandwiches, fresh fruits, carrot and celery sticks, saltless pretzels, rice cakes, bagels, and air-popped popcorn?

Mini Meals And Exercise: The Dynamic Duo

Perhaps the greatest advantage of eating small meals is that they don't bloat you and cause paralyzing fatigue. After a feast, you're lucky if you can keep your eyes open, much less engage in any sort of calorie-burning activity.

Not so with small meals, which can actually leave you feeling energized and therefore likely to do something a little more physical than collapsing in front of the TV.

This important but often overlooked point touches on something critical to the weight-loss process. Large meals encourage the inactivity that allows calories to be stored as fat. Small meals, on the other hand, energize you and stimulate the physical activity needed to burn calories for energy.

Better yet, studies show that physical activity within 30 minutes of eating is an especially good way to burn calories—in fact it's 10 percent better than exercising on an empty stomach. The scientific term for this phenomenon is the "thermal effect of food," which can amount to a sizable weight loss advantage over time. Simply by taking a short walk after just one mini meal a day, you could make significant progress in reaching your weight-loss goals.

When "Life" Weighs Too Much: Can Too Much Stress Make You Fat?

If you think it's too much food combined with too little exercise that makes us fat, you might want to think again. According to research presented in 1994 at the International Conference on Obesity, stress can be fattening. During times of anxiety—whether during a traffic jam or an argument with a co-worker—your body produces adrenaline, a hormone that increases the heart rate and causes molecules of fat to be released into your bloodstream. This gives you the energy needed to deal with the stressful situation.

So what do we do instead?

Instead of getting physical, we get frustrated and begin to "stew." This causes our bodies to produce another hormone called cortisol, which acts as a kind of peacemaker to help the fighting-mad fat molecules get reabsorbed. Unfortunately, cortisol helps other fat molecules get absorbed, too, specifically in the stomach area. It seems unfair and illogical, but numerous studies have proven that it does happen. In a study at Wake Forest University in Winston-Salem, North Carolina, monkeys subjected to chronic stress had significantly more fat in the area of their abdomens than monkeys allowed to live stress free.

"Chronic stress plays a role in abdominal fat distribution," remarked Robert K. Cooper, Ph.D., in his book *Low-Fat Living* (Rodale Press, 1996). "The more minutes of each day you are frustrated, impatient, or angry, the more likely that stress is contributing to fat-making in your body."

Add the overeating we tend to do when we're stressed—usually high-fat junk foods—and the "fret more, weigh more" picture becomes all too clear.

Try These Techniques to Reduce
Stress Instantly!

The experts recommend combating stress immediately. The sooner the better, in fact, because the faster stress is defused, the less it's apt to accumulate in ways that can become physically harmful. Here are some clinically proven techniques for reducing stress the moment it strikes.

Breathe stress away. When stress strikes, our first reaction is to halt our breathing entirely for several seconds or more, and then to breathe quickly and shallowly. This reduces oxygen to the brain, which makes us feel stressed even more. To prevent this, it's important to make a conscious effort to breathe deeply and slowly at the first signs of stress. Inhale slowly but deeply through your nose so that your abdomen expands first, then your chest. Then exhale slowly through your mouth, imagining the stress leaving your body as you do.

Think relaxing thoughts. Most stressful situations are beyond our control, which is precisely why we find them stressful. It can be helpful, therefore, to divorce yourself as much as possible from the cause of your stress, thinking totally unrelated and pleasant thoughts, instead. If you're caught in a traffic jam, for example, or find yourself waiting in what seems like an endless line, think of your favorite vacation spot, or a romantic encounter with your sweetheart!

Sharpen your sense of humor. Often the only difference between a stressful situation and a humorous one lies in how we view it. The trash bag that breaks and spills its contents on your newly waxed kitchen floor. The sweater that your daughter converts from a size 12 to a 6 by mistakenly putting it in the dryer. Whether such events are tragedies or comedies is entirely up to you, and the sooner you realize that, the less stressful they're going to be.

Don't take things personally. The stock market takes a plunge. The price of gasoline goes up. It's only natural to view such events in terms of how they affect us personally. But to do so is not only highly stressful, it's self-centered and inaccurate as well. Life's inconveniences affect us all, so we should stop feeling persecuted when they occur.

Get physical. Research shows that physical activity can help stop stress the moment it strikes. In addition, people who are physically active are better at coping with stressful events in the first place. So take a walk, play tennis, go for a jog, or ride a bike the next time life's burdens seem too heavy to bear. The "strength" you gain will lighten your load, both immediately and in the long run.

Open up to loved ones or friends. When stress mounts, it needs an outlet or it will fester and grow. Talk with the people who are closest to you when you're feeling stressed. Not only will this make you feel better, it will tighten your bond with these people, thus ensuring an emotional oasis for the future.

Cook a healthful, low-fat meal. Just because stress is often accompanied by an urge to eat doesn't mean this urge has to be bad. If you can get your mind off your problems by preparing a fantastic, four-star, low-fat feast, that urge to eat can be decidedly healthful!

FAT-BURNING FACT:

Lunch meats are among the fattiest meats and one of the top sources of fat in the American diet. The most healthful choices are boiled ham, honey loaf, and turkey breast.

CHAPTER 3

HOW FITNESS FIGHTS FAT

So where does exercise fit into the fat-burning picture?

Smack dab in the middle. In fact, exercise is essential to the fat-burning process because it infuses our bodies with the very component that fat-burning relies on most: oxygen. This is especially true of aerobic exercise, which "fans the flames" of the fat-burning process. Aerobic exercise can increase your body's uptake of oxygen by as much as 20 times—enough to create quite a fat "bonfire." The more fit you become, moreover, the better your body gets at making sure fat cells become the target of this oxygen rush.

But as great as aerobic exercise is, its appetite for calories can actually be increased if combined with exercises like strength training. Strength training not only exercises your current muscle cells, it helps create new ones, resulting in more "cylinders" in your fat-burning engine. Better yet, muscle tissue is metabolically active even at rest. By adding strength training to your exercise routine, you increase the rate at which you burn calories—not just as you're exercising but as you're sleeping or watching TV!

This is why study after study has shown what every couch potato hates to hear most: People who are the most successful at losing weight and keeping it off are the ones who include at least some form of exercise in their weight-control efforts.

Exercise is crucial to successful weight loss, not just because of the number of calories it burns but because of the *type* of calories it burns. If done regularly and in the right ways (which we'll be seeing shortly), exercise can actually teach your body to burn calories from fat even more so than from carbohydrates. Exercise does this by encouraging the formation of enzymes that make fat more available as fuel for muscular activity. Once these enzymes begin to work their fat-burning "magic," you'll begin to have more energy. You'll start burning more calories at everything you do, whether it's vacuuming the living room or spending an afternoon in the park with your kids.

Give Yourself a Break:
Take It Easy

Exercise is a fat cell's worst nightmare, and that's great. But there are barely enough hours in your day as it is, and you're supposed to find time to work out?

Relax. Exercise need not be as torturous or time-consuming as some fitness experts would like us to believe. In fact, the latest research has found that substantial health benefits can be gained by moderate activities adding up to as little as 150 calories worth of energy expenditure a day.

And please notice we said "add up." Contrary to the belief that exercise must be continuous for at least 20 to 30 minutes to do any good, research shows that you can exercise for shorter periods of time and still reap the benefits. In one study at the University of Pittsburgh, for example, researchers found that women who walked for 40 minutes a day in separate 10-minute sessions enjoyed the same health benefits and actually lost more weight than women who walked for 40 minutes continuously. "The greater flexibility associated with exercising in short bouts evidently had helped the women to be more consistent in their exercise participation," remarked the researchers in their report in the *International Journal of Obesity.*

FAT-BURNING FACT:

A study by the YMCA found that people who lifted weights three times a week for just 20 minutes gained 6 pounds of muscle and lost 15 pounds of fat in just seven weeks.

So, yes, you can be fit and keep a busy schedule, too! All you need to do is find ways to get your exercise in manageable "nibbles" rather than in those inconvenient (and easily skipped) half-hour chunks. A short walk here, a quick bike ride there, and maybe some gardening or housework in between. As long as these activities add up to at least 150 calories of energy expended each day, you're giving your body's metabolism the fat-burning boost that long-term weight control requires.

This is not to say that more exercise cannot burn more calories and therefore more unwanted fat, but an energy expenditure of approximately 150 calories a day is a healthful and reasonable start—especially if you're relatively new to the fitness game. If you choose to pursue an exercise program more avidly, fine. Just be sure to check first with your doctor, and consider consulting a licensed fitness expert on how best to proceed to achieve your desired goals.

Strength Training: Burning Fat by Building Muscle

The key to burning calories is movement. The good news is that the movement doesn't have to be continuous or so strenuous that you find yourself gasping for breath. Studies now show that exercise that's too strenuous—by putting the body into a state of oxygen deficit—can actually shut fat-burning down. You need plenty of oxygen, which is what you will get when you exercise aerobically, to get the fat "going." By exercising so vigorously that you force yourself into an oxygen shortage, you cause your body to switch from burning fat to burning glycogen. Glycogen is a form of carbohydrate stored in the muscles and liver that the body can use for energy with virtually no oxygen at all.

But as mentioned at the beginning of this chapter, there's another type of exercise that can boost fat burning to an even higher level, and that's strength training—the kind that builds muscle. This isn't to say that aerobic exercise isn't an invaluable weight-control aid, because it most certainly is, as dozens of studies show. But the primary value of aerobic exercise lies in its ability to burn calories as you're actually in the process of doing it, which to a degree limits its weight-control value. This is not the case with strength training, which, because it builds muscle, can make you a better calorie burner 24 hours a day, even as you're talking on the phone or relaxing in a nice warm bath. (Some studies have shown that very long and strenuous aerobic workouts also can be followed by a period of increased calorie burning, but usually this lasts no more than several hours.)

FAT-BURNING FACT:

A "rep" is short for "repetition." A "set" is a group of repetitions. Two "sets" of eight "reps," therefore, would be two groups of an exercise performed eight times, making sixteen in all.

The Proof in the Pudding

As proof of the fat-burning power of strength training, consider the following study done recently with seventy-two men and women at the YMCA in Quincy, Massachusetts. Half of the people worked out aerobically for 30 minutes three times a week, while the other group split their workouts between 15 minutes of aerobics and 15 minutes of lifting weights. Both groups had identical meals (consisting of 60 percent carbohydrates, 20 percent protein, and 20 percent fat), and yet results differed dramatically. The strength-training group had lost an impressive 10 pounds of fat over the course of the eight-week study, while the aerobics group had lost only three.

Sounds great, you say, but you don't want bulky muscles, even if they are such great fat-blasters?

You don't have to have bulky muscles. You can appreciably raise your body's basal metabolism (the rate at which you burn calories at rest) simply by toning and strengthening the muscles you already have. It's important that you do this because studies show that the muscle mass of the average American woman decreases by about a half a pound a year after the age of 35— enough to cause a considerable slow-down in metabolic rate and significant accumulations of unwanted fat.

A Little Goes a Long Way

"This is one of the reasons for the seemingly mysterious weight gain so many of us experience as we get older," says Bryant Stamford, of the Center for Health Promotion at the University of Louisville. "Even though we don't eat any more, and we keep our activity levels basically the same, we gain weight because we lose muscle mass and hence our ability to burn calories at a more youthful rate."

But how much strength training is required to stall this loss of muscle tissue associated with aging? Will you need to be setting up a gym in your garage?

As with aerobic exercise, there's good news here, too. Studies show that age-related muscle loss can be decreased significantly with weight-training sessions or strength-building exercises, such as push-ups and pull-ups, done as infrequently as twice a week. Better yet, many chores around the house also can keep your muscles toned and metabolism perked. Raking leaves, carrying firewood, scrubbing floors, moving furniture, shoveling snow, carrying grocery bags, kneading bread, or toting around a toddler or two. Any activity that pits muscles against some form of resistance—whether it's a barbell or basket of wet laundry—can be an effective way to keep muscle cells functioning at their fat-burning best.

Fitness And Soap Operas

If you're like most Americans, your number one excuse for not getting more exercise is lack of time, yet you still manage to watch an average of 4 hours of television a day. So why not combine the two? By spending just 30 minutes doing some form of light exercise, such as riding a stationary bike or walking on a treadmill while viewing the tube, you could be 20 pounds thinner this time next year.

"I'm convinced that strength training has been the missing link in many peoples' weight-control efforts up to this point, and especially people over the age of about 40," Dr. Stamford says. "Middle age is when muscle-building hormones begin their greatest decline, and yet few of us respond by doing the kind of strength training needed to compensate for it. Usually we'll take up an aerobic activity such as walking or cycling as we age, thus missing out on the opportunity to keep our muscles—and metabolisms—as well toned as they could be."

This is not to say that we can halt the loss of muscle tissue entirely as we age. But take a look at legendary fitness guru Jack LaLanne, who, to celebrate his 65th birthday, swam across a 1 1/2-mile lake pulling 65 rowboats loaded with 65,000 pounds of wood pulp—while handcuffed! It's pretty clear that many of us are letting Father Time take more of our muscle power—and our ability to burn calories—than necessary.

How Active Are You?
Take a Minute to Take This Test

The good news from the Centers for Disease Control and Prevention (CDC) is that we don't have to burden ourselves with continuous 20- to 30-minute aerobic workouts to enjoy the health benefits of exercise. Instead, any combination of moderate activities adding up to an average of at least 150 calories of energy expenditure a day is the new recommendation for helping us avoid the pitfalls (increased risks of heart disease, diabetes, osteoporosis, depression, and certain forms of cancer) of a sedentary lifestyle.

But before you sit down on the couch to celebrate that less exhaustive prescription, you might want to take an honest look at the amount of physical activity your average day actually includes. We offer the following quiz to help you do just that.

1. **In an average day, I climb the following number of flights of stairs (12 steps per flight):**

   a. 0   (0 points)
   b. 1–5   (1 point)
   c. 6–10   (2 points)
   d. more than 10   (4 points)

2. **My job requires that I be on my feet and moving for approximately the following number of hours per day:**

   a. 0 hours   (0 points)
   b. 1 hour   (2 points)

c. 2 hours   (3 points)
d. 3 hours   (4 points)
e. 4 hours or more   (6 points)

3. My job requires heavy labor such as lifting, carrying, shoveling, or climbing for the following number of hours a day:

a. 0 hours   (0 points)
b. 1 hour   (3 points)
c. 2 hours   (5 points)
d. 3 hours   (7 points)
e. 4 hours   (9 points)
f. 5 hours or more   (12 points)

4. I spend the following number of hours a week tending a garden or lawn. (Points assume activity is year-round. Cut points in half if activity is seasonal.)

a. 0 hours   (0 points)
b. 1 hour   (1 point)
c. 2 hours   (2 points)
d. 3 hours   (3 points)
e. 4 hours   (4 points)
f. 5 hours or more   (6 points)

5. I participate in light sporting activities or dancing for the following number of hours a week:

a. 0 hours   (0 points)
b. 1 hour   (1 point)
c. 2 hours   (2 points)
d. 3 hours   (3 points)
e. 4 or more hours   (4 points)

6. I try to walk for the following distance most days of the week:

a. 0 miles   (0 points)
b. 1 mile   (2 points)
c. 2 miles   (4 points)
d. 3 miles   (6 points)
e. 4 miles or more   (10 points)

7. I spend the following number of hours each week doing household chores such as cleaning, dusting, vacuuming, or laundry:

a. 0 hours   (0 points)
b. 1 hour   (1 point)
c. 2 hours   (2 points)
d. 3 hours   (3 points)
e. 4 hours   (4 points)
f. more than 4 hours   (6 points)

8. I engage in some form of aerobic exercise (i.e., jogging, cycling, swimming, fast-walking, aerobic dancing, or working out on a rowing machine or stair-climber) for the following number of hours a week:

a. 0 hours   (0 points)
b. 1 hour   (5 points)
c. 2 hours   (10 points)
d. 3 hours   (15 points)
e. more than 3 hours   (20 points)

9. I participate in strength-building exercise (by lifting free weights, working out on weight machines, or doing strength-building calisthenics such as chin-ups and push-ups) for the following number of hours each week:

a. 0 hours   (0 points)
b. 1 hour   (5 points)
c. 2 hours   (10 points)
d. 3 hours   (15 points)
e. more than 3 hours   (20 points)

10. I am a parent in charge of taking care of one or more preschool-aged children for the following amount of time each day:

a. children home all day (5 points)
b. children home half a day
   (day-care center the rest) (3 points)
c. children spend all day at day-care center (1 point)

SCORING

15 points or higher: Superb. Congratulations! You're getting more exercise than are approximately 80 percent of your fellow Americans. If you also are eating well, not smoking, avoiding undue stress, and drinking in moderation only, you're doing all you can to live a long and productive life.

10–14 points: Very Good. Nice work. You're doing what's required to satisfy your basic exercise needs. If you're also adhering to the other healthful behaviors mentioned above, your life should be long and prosperous.

5–9 points: Marginal. You're not to be scolded but not commended either. By fitting more activity into your life, you could be slimmer, have more energy, and also improve your chances of living longer.

Less than 5 points: Reprehensible! You're a member of the Couch Potato Hall of Fame and had better check your pulse frequently. Your level of inactivity is hazardous to your health and waistline, too.

Shape Up Your Metabolism In Just 30 Minutes A Week

Strength training can really put a "squeeze" on fat cells. By building and toning muscle tissue, it can make you a better calorie-burner 24 hours a day. Better yet, you don't have to become an iron-pumping fanatic to do it. All you need is to put your major muscle groups up against some form of resistance for approximately 15 minutes at least two to three times a week. Chores around the house and yard can qualify as strength-building exercises (scrubbing floors, moving furniture, digging in the garden, and trimming hedges and trees, for example). If such activities are not available to you, or you'd like something more regimented, try a simple weight-training program (see below) or maybe some strength-building calisthenics, such as push-ups and pull-ups, to give your muscles a major fat-burning boost.

The Six Greatest Fat-burning Muscle Groups— And How To Work Them All In Just 20 Minutes!

The physics principle of calorie burning is this: The larger the muscle group, the more calories it will burn. The key to strength training for weight control is to work the largest muscles you have (listed below). Also listed are the best exercises for getting these muscles into the maximum, fat-burning shape.

And don't think you'll need a lot of expensive equipment, or that you'll have to spend grueling hours at the gym. You can maximize the fat-burning power of all your major muscle groups by using just dumbbells, and you'll only need about 20 minutes, three times a week. Certainly you can find time for that, right?

How Much To Lift

You'll want to do this series of six exercises twice, with a rest period between each series lasting one to two minutes. As for the exercises themselves, do "sets" consisting of 10 repetitions each, using a weight that is heavy enough so that your tenth "rep" is difficult but not torturous. After completing each set of 10 reps, take about a 15- to 30-second rest before moving on to the next set. The entire workout should take only about 20 minutes.

The Muscle Group	The Exercise
Chest	Dumbbell bench presses, or push-ups
Thighs	Squats
Shoulders and Back	Reverse dumbbell "flys" or pull-ups
Biceps	Dumbbell curls
Triceps	Dumbbell presses
Abdomen	Curl-ups

Making The Fitness Fit

Beginning to get the picture? Exercise—a combination of aerobic and strength-building exercise, especially—trains the body to favor fat as an energy source. Better yet, the amount and type of exercise required to do this is well within reach of all of us, even working mothers with barely a minute to spare. "Many of us could get all the exercise we need if we'd simply stop trying so hard to avoid it," says Dr. Bryant Stamford.

But, no, we take elevators instead of stairs, and drive around endlessly to find the most convenient parking spot, and buy every device imaginable to make our household chores and yard work easier. Or worse yet, we'll avoid our physical chores entirely by hiring them out to professionals. A recent Gallup poll showed that we spend an average of over $700 a year per household on lawn-care services alone. We're burning our money when we could be burning calories!

And compounding this absurdity is the fact that millions of us join health clubs—which we fail to visit—in hopes of getting the very exercise we've gone to so much trouble to avoid! "We've made exercise far more complicated, impractical, and inconvenient than it has to be, so no wonder only about a third of us currently get the amount of exercise we need," Dr. Stamford says. "We need to learn to incorporate exercise into our lives in ways that are more enjoyable and practical."

Exercise For The Health Of It

Exercise is just what the doctor ordered for achieving and maintaining a healthy weight. Exercise also is just what the doctor ordered for achieving a healthy body, something ancient healers have known since the writings of Hippocrates. Studies now show that 30 minutes of moderate exercise a day, in addition to keeping your metabolism in the best fat-burning shape, also can bestow the following important health benefits:

- Improved circulation (achieved through the widening of existing blood vessels plus the formation of new ones) resulting in reduced risks of heart attacks and strokes

- Lower blood pressure resulting in reduced risks of aneurysms (an abnormal blood-filled swelling of a blood vessel), glaucoma, heart attacks, and strokes

- Reductions in "bad" (LDL) and increases in "good" (HDL) cholesterol resulting in reduced risks of clogged arteries leading to heart attacks and strokes

- Reduced risks of adult-onset (type 2) diabetes

- Increased physical as well as mental stamina

- Stronger bones resulting in reduced risks of osteoporosis

- Improved joint mobility resulting in reduced risks of osteoarthritis

- A stronger immune system resulting in reduced risks of colds, flu, and possibly even cancer

- Improved digestion resulting in the best absorption of vital nutrients

- Reduced risks of low-back pain

- An increase in the blood's ability to carry oxygen to cells, plus an increase in the ability of muscle cells to use this oxygen to burn fat

- An increase in the blood's ability to rid the body of carbon dioxide and other cellular waste products

- Greater intestinal regularity resulting in reduced risks of cancer of the colon

- Sounder, more restful sleep

- Healthier skin

- Reduced risks of depression and anxiety disorders

- Protection from stress

- More enjoyable sex

Exercise For A Slimmer Appetite

But with all the calories exercise burns, won't it just make you eat more, thus canceling all the exercise's fantastic weight-control benefits?

No. In fact, just the opposite tends to be true. In addition to burning calories, exercise can actually help reduce your urge to take in calories in the first place. "Many people who embark on fitness programs are surprised to find that it actually helps them eat less, not more," says Dr. Stamford.

As evidence of this, he cites a study done several years ago in which people reported feeling less hungry and more energetic several hours after taking a 15-minute walk than they did after eating a candy bar. "The tendency of exercise to reduce appetite probably stems from its ability to mobilize supplies of blood sugar, called glycogen, which is stored in the muscles and the liver," says Dr. Stamford.

Then, too, there are the psychological benefits of exercise that can help keep runaway appetites in check: improvements in self-esteem and self-control and increased abilities to cope with stress, for example. "When people exercise regularly, they often find they feel more in control of every other aspect of their lives—their work, their relationships, and their diets, especially," says Dr. Stamford. "Exercise can be a very powerful catalyst for all sorts of healthful behaviors. Studies show it can even help people give up smoking."

FAT-BURNING FACT:

The amount of refined sugar consumed by the average American adult in a single day: 20 teaspoons.

Every Little Bit Counts

But what about "no pain, no gain"? Can activities that are fun or useful be strenuous enough to do us any good?

Absolutely. "The latest research now shows that exercise is pretty much a case of anything goes," says Stanford University sports medicine specialist Warren Scott, M.D. "As long as it's bodily movement, it qualifies as exercise, and it's clearly better than no activity at all. We know now, too, that exercise that's gotten in bits and pieces can be as beneficial as exercise gotten in larger and more onerous chunks. Exercise does not have to have you huffing and puffing for at least 20 continuous minutes to do you any good, which is the impression, unfortunately, that many people still have."

Look over the activities on the next page with that in mind. They all burn at least 150 calories, the amount that research now indicates is needed to satisfy our minimum daily exercise requirements. If you've got the time or inclination to do more, that's fine. Just don't make the mistake of doing no exercise because you don't think you have the time to do enough. Remember, the latest research shows that any amount of exercise is vastly better than none at all.

More Gain, Less Pain
50 Fun and Practical Ways
to Burn 150 Calories in 30 Minutes or Less

Not the jogging or iron-pumping type? No problem. There are plenty of other more enjoyable and practical ways to burn off unwanted pounds, as the following list shows. Your goal, remember, is to burn at least 150 calories by engaging in any of these activities each day. (Calorie expenditures are for someone weighing 150 pounds. Adjust figures up or down slightly if you weigh more or less.)

Activity	Calories Burned In 30 Minutes
Backpacking	280
Basketball (shooting baskets)	180
Basketball (playing in game)	320
Bicycling (leisurely)	160
Bicycling (vigorously)	400
Canoeing (moderate effort)	280
Dancing (ballroom or disco)	220
Dancing (aerobic, low-impact)	240
Dancing (aerobic, high-impact)	280
Fishing (from stream, in wading boots)	160
Football (touch)	320
Golf (pulling clubs)	200
Hackysack	160
Handball	480
Hockey (field)	320
Hockey (ice)	320
Horseback riding (trot)	260
Horseback riding (gallop)	320

Horse grooming	240
Housework (sweeping, mopping, etc.)	180
Hunting (small game)	200
Ice skating (recreational)	280
In-line skating (moderately fast)	280
Jumping rope (moderately fast)	400
Karate (or other martial arts class)	400
Moving furniture (heavy)	360
Painting (outdoors)	200
Ping-Pong	160
Playing with children (vigorous)	200
Playing drums	160
Rock climbing	440
Scuba diving	280
Skateboarding	200
Skiing, downhill (moderate effort)	240
Skiing, cross-country (moderate effort)	340
Sledding (or tobogganing)	280
Snorkeling	200
Snowshoeing (moderate effort)	320
Soccer	360
Softball (pitching)	240
Squash	480
Swimming (freestyle, moderate effort)	320
Tai chi	160
Tennis (singles)	320
Tennis (doubles)	240
Volleyball (beach)	320
Walking (moderate pace)	150
Walking (brisk pace)	180
Water polo	400
Water skiing	240

Fitness On The Mild Side: The Case of Robert

"I used to really hate my workouts, which might help explain why I was so good at missing them," Robert now confesses. "I'd push myself to the limit every time, thinking I wasn't doing myself any good if I didn't. Then I'd sometimes go a week or more without working out at all, because the whole experience was so dreadful for me."

Not just dreadful but unproductive. Robert was about 20 pounds overweight with high blood pressure and a high serum cholesterol level, but his sporadic workouts were having very little effect.

Not only was he failing to lose weight, his cholesterol level and blood pressure were inching upward, "the result, probably, of all the stress I was subjecting myself to," he now says. "I was under tremendous pressure at work, and I think my approach to exercise was probably only adding to it. Either I was dreading my workouts, or feeling guilty for avoiding them, certainly not a very relaxing situation either way."

But as fate would have it, Robert was "saved" one day by an injury. He tore a muscle in his left calf—"the result of going out too fast without adequately warming up," his doctor told him—and was forced to modify his fitness regime. On his doctor's advice, he started walking. Before long he actually started to like it.

"It was a whole different experience," Robert says. "I stopped worrying about how fast I was going, or how far, and just let my mind wander. I started liking it so much, in fact, that I actually began looking forward to it as a way of unwinding after work. I even started inviting my wife along, and we'd have some really great talks."

Better yet, Robert's weight started to come down, along with his blood pressure and cholesterol levels. "I've even started to take a slightly more relaxed approach to my work," he says. "I don't see things so much as just black or white anymore, and I don't think I'm as impulsive or critical. It's as though I've slowed down the revs of my engine, and yet I actually feel more productive."

How To "Excuse-Proof" Your Exercise Routine

But you already know that exercise is good for you, and you want to do it. The problem you have is sticking to a regular schedule. Something always seems to come up that gets in the way. Then you need to make exercise more of a priority, says Kerry Courneya, Ph.D., of the University of Calgary in Alberta, Canada. Here are some tips that can help:

1. **Choose an activity you enjoy.** The reason you're finding excuses not to exercise is probably because you don't like whatever it is you're doing. As we mentioned earlier in this chapter, exercise does not have to be strenuous to work. So go easy on yourself and have fun with your exercise. Take scenic walks, play tennis, play frisbee with the kids. Remember, anything that gets you moving is going to burn calories. It's sitting around feeling guilty for not doing anything at all that can get fattening.

2. **Try to exercise before you begin your day.** Studies show that people who exercise first thing in the morning are less likely to skip their workouts than people who wait until later in the day, when other obligations pop up and get in the way. Remember, too, that exercise is a great energizer and spirit-lifter, so you'll be all the more ready to face the world by working out before you begin your day.

3. **Involve friends.** Not only is it harder to skip workouts when you involve others, exercising with friends also can make the experience a lot more fun.

4. **Reward yourself.** There's nothing like putting occasional "pots" at the end of your exercise rainbow to keep you going, says psychologist James Prochaska, Ph.D., of the University of Rhode Island. If you've succeeded in sticking to a schedule you've set up for yourself, go ahead and do something nice for yourself periodically, he says. A new dress, a dinner out, some new running shoes, perhaps.

3. **Don't get derailed if you do miss.** It's inevitable that even the most dedicated exercisers get knocked off course occasionally—so why shouldn't you? Just remember that it's the "big picture" that's important and get back on track as soon as you can. The worst thing to do is to become immobilized with guilt.

Look Before You Leap Into A Health Club

Should you join a health club or gym to help solidify your exercise commitment?

That depends on you—and the club. For some people, the structure and camaraderie provided by a fitness facility can be very motivating. For others it can be a source of stress that only makes exercising even more burdensome.

If you think you would be more comfortable with the former than the latter, then by all means go for it. But do some investigating before signing on any dotted lines. Visit the facility, of course, but also ask the following questions of the management:

- **What, exactly, does a membership include?** The facility should offer a free fitness evaluation, plus a session with an instructor, to get you started on a program designed specifically for you.

- **Can your membership be refunded or sold to someone else?** Many clubs will allow this if you are dissatisfied.

- **Are discounts available for using the club during off-hours?** Some clubs offer reduced rates for mid-morning hours and afternoons during the week.

- **What qualifications do the instructors have?** Be wary of a facility whose instructors have no formal training at all.

- **Is the facility's equipment leased or owned?** Leasing is preferable because it means the equipment will more likely be kept up-to-date.

- Will there be hours when any of the club's facilities are unavailable because of special classes or workouts by local teams? Swimming pools sometimes get reserved for this reason.

- Does the club demand a down payment before you've had a chance to read the contract? If so, take your fitness somewhere else.

Last but not least, visit the facility and chat with some of its members. If they have any gripes, chances are you will, too.

Walking: Possibly The Best Exercise Of All

Nothing against all that new fitness equipment available today—everything from stair-climbers to cardio-gliders—but one of the most effective and practical forms of exercise to burn fat continues to be walking. As Mark Bricklin, the former editor of *Prevention* magazine, says, "No other activity bestows the blessings of exercise as easily, enjoyably, and safely as the simple act of going for a walk."

That might sound like a pretty lofty claim, but there's a lot of research to back it up. Studies show that people who walk for fitness suffer the fewest injuries, have the lowest dropout rates, and continue to exercise later in life more than people who exercise in any other way.

The "Leader Of The Pack" For Weight Control

When it comes to weight control, walking really jumps out ahead of the pack. In one study done at the University of California Medical Center, a group of obese people who repeatedly had failed to lose weight by dieting lost an average of 22 pounds in a year simply by walking for 30 minutes a day. "The key to walking seems to be that it's one of the few activities people will do with the consistency that long-term weight loss requires," Bricklin says. "People usually will exercise more frequently and for longer periods of time when they walk, and that translates into more calories burned."

Could walking be your best fitness and fat-burning route? Why not give it a try and find out for yourself? Here are some general guidelines for getting started:

Wear proper shoes.

And no, this does not mean running shoes. They will do in a pinch, but it's best if you wear shoes specifically designed for walking.

Don't be in too great a hurry.

Your goal should be at least 30 minutes a day, but feel free to take as long as a month to reach that goal if your current fitness level is low.

Put consistency ahead of distance or speed.

You're better off walking a little every day than going for longer or faster walks with several days of rest in between.

Try to walk after meals.

Studies show that this can boost the amount of calories you burn by as much as 10 percent.

Use proper form.

You've been walking since the age of approximately 18 months, so you think you've got it down. But don't be so sure. To obtain the best health benefits from your walks:

1. Walk with your back straight, your chin up, and your arms swinging freely at your sides while bent at a 90-degree angle.

2. Do not walk flat-footed. Push off from the balls of your feet and land on your heels.

3. Lean slightly forward and pump harder with your arms when walking up hills.

4. To walk faster, quicken your movement rather than lengthen your steps.

5. Breathe deeply and with a rhythm that feels comfortably in sync with your stride.

A word on walking with weights: Sorry, but studies show they do not appreciably boost calorie-burning as you walk, although they can help tone the muscles of the arms. (Weights weighing between 2 and 3 pounds but no more than 5 pounds are best.) Ankle weights, on the other hand, are not a good idea. Research shows they can increase risks of injury by altering foot placement and stride.

Patience and Realism

So now you know how to eat and exercise your way to a leaner and healthier body. Two things you should try to remember along the way: (1) The longer your weight loss takes, the longer it's apt to last, and (2) Do not strive for a weight that is unrealistically low. Our best "fighting" weights, research has begun to discover, usually are within a range we don't have to fight.

Good Luck!

CHAPTER 4

VITAMINS AND MINERALS

BEST FOOD SOURCES

There's more to food than just protein, carbohydrates, fat, and calories. Food also contains vitamins and minerals—and it's a good thing, too, because you couldn't live without them! Vitamins work as "catalysts," meaning that they help produce the chemical reactions required for your body to put food to proper use. Minerals, in a slightly different way, help provide the right "environment" so that these chemical reactions can happen as they should. Together, vitamins and minerals—a little like Batman and Robin—work as a "dynamic duo."

VITAMINS

VITAMIN A

Vitamin A is appropriately named because it deserves an "A" for its stellar contributions to good health. In addition to playing a vital role in good vision, it contributes to healthy skin, aids in the production of red blood cells, and helps keep the body's immune system in shape. It may even help prevent cancer. Among other foods, Vitamin A is found in:

- Cantaloupe
- Carrots
- Liver (all types)
- Mangoes
- Pumpkin
- Spinach
- Sweet potatoes
- Turnip greens
- Winter squash

THE B VITAMINS

The B vitamins act as your body's spark plugs. They help derive energy from carbohydrates and can be found most abundantly in the following:

- Beans
- Brewer's yeast
- Brown rice
- Eggs
- Liver
- Meats
- Milk
- Nuts
- Whole grains

VITAMIN C

Vitamin C's most critical function is to help the body ward off not just colds but infections in general. The following are excellent sources of Vitamin C:

- Broccoli
- Brussels sprouts
- Cantaloupe
- Citrus fruits
- Currants
- Honeydew melon
- Kiwi fruit
- Kohlrabi (cabbage turnip)
- Red peppers
- Strawberries

VITAMIN D

Your body manufactures bone-building Vitamin D, called the "sunshine vitamin," when exposed to sunlight. Because this can be a problem during cold weather, which keeps us indoors, it's important to get enough D in your diet. The best way to do that is to drink plenty of Vitamin D-fortified low-fat or skim milk. No other foods, unfortunately, contain the vitamin in appreciable amounts.

VITAMIN E

Think of Vitamin E as your body's "enforcer." It helps other essential vitamins work better at protecting you from everything from the common cold to cancer. Because the best food sources of Vitamin E tend also to be quite high in fat (vegetable oils and nuts, for example), many nutritionists recommend a daily supplement of approximately 100 to 400 International Units (IUs) of Vitamin E. Other sources:

- Blackberries
- Corn oil
- Hazelnut oil
- Mangoes
- Mayonnaise
- Olive oil
- Safflower oil
- Sunflower oil
- Wheat germ

MINERALS

CALCIUM

Calcium is a mineral with several important functions: It helps strengthen our bones, it stabilizes our blood pressure, and it helps maintain a healthy heart. Thankfully, calcium is found in many foods, including:

- Broccoli
- Low-fat and nonfat cheeses
- Low-fat and nonfat milk
- Low-fat and nonfat yogurt
- Salmon
- Sardines
- Tofu
- Turnip greens
- Soybeans

IRON

The primary function of iron—and it's a critical one—is to assure that the body manufactures enough hemoglobin, a protein that helps red blood cells transport oxygen to virtually every tissue of the body. Iron also plays an important role in keeping the body's immune system functioning properly, so it's important that our diets include enough of this mineral. The best source of iron is meat, but it also can be found, in a less absorbable form, in plant foods. Because meat can be high in fat, most nutritionists recommend getting iron from a good mix of both meat and non-meat sources. Iron is found in the following foods:

- Beef
- Blackstrap molasses
- Chicken
- Clams
- Leafy green vegetables
- Liver (all types)
- Oysters
- Pork
- Potatoes
- Soybeans
- Tofu
- Whole grains

MAGNESIUM

Magnesium is another "multi-purpose" mineral, important for the health of bones, blood vessels, the heart, and the immune system. It is present in many foods, the best of which are:

- Almonds
- Brown or wild rice
- Cashew nuts
- Halibut
- Mackerel
- Pumpkin seeds
- Spinach
- Sunflower seeds
- Tofu
- Wheat germ

POTASSIUM

Potassium's main function seems to be to help control blood pressure, but new research shows that it also may help prevent strokes and kidney stones, too. People who exercise heavily may need ample amounts of potassium to prevent muscle cramps. Look to these foods as your best potassium sources:

- Avocadoes
- Bananas
- Cantaloupe
- Clams
- Dried apricots
- Lima beans
- Nonfat yogurt
- Oranges
- Potatoes
- Rainbow trout
- Raisins
- Skim milk
- Yams

ZINC

Zinc is the key to a healthy immune system and to healthy (more wrinkle-resistant) skin. As the following list shows, meat products (aside from shellfish) tend to be the richest source of zinc, so try to get your zinc from the leanest cuts when possible. (Zinc requirements will increase during pregnancy, so moms-to-be, take note.)

- Beans
- Beef
- Clams
- Crabmeat
- Liver (most types)
- Nonfat yogurt
- Oysters
- Peas
- Salmon
- Wild rice
- Wheat germ
- Whole grains

The Sense—And Nonsense—of Supplements

If vitamins and minerals are so important for good health, should you be taking supplements to be even healthier? Unless you're over the age of approximately 60 (when the body's ability to absorb nutrients begins to decline), or you're on a strict, very low-calorie diet (which you shouldn't be without the supervision of your doctor), taking more than the current RDA (Recommended Dietary Allowance) of most vitamins and minerals shouldn't be necessary—and in some cases can even be harmful, the experts say. Only Vitamin E is difficult to get in adequate amounts through food, hence a daily supplement of 100 to 400 IUs often is recommend. "There's no question that nutrients are better absorbed when gotten through foods," says vitamin expert Ronald Watson, Ph.D., of the University of Arizona. "Food also contains a wide variety of micronutrients, the benefits of which we're just beginning to understand."

And there's another reason: Healthful foods beat vitamin pills in the taste department every time!

CHAPTER 5

NICE AND EASY FAT-BURNING RECIPES

Simply Delicious Soups and Salads

Onion-Potato Soup

1	tablespoon canola, corn, safflower, or sunflower oil
2	large onions, chopped
2	teaspoons all-purpose flour
1	cup beef broth or bouillon
1	large potato, peeled, and cut into 1/2-inch pieces
1/4	cup frozen peas
2 1/2	cups skim milk
1/2	teaspoon salt
	pepper to taste

Heat oil in Dutch oven or large saucepan over high heat; add onions. Cook 5 to 7 minutes or until onions just begin to brown. Reduce heat to medium. Stir in flour. Gradually stir in beef broth, then add potato and peas. Cover and cook until potato is tender, about 15 to 20 minutes, stirring occasionally to get up brown bits. In food processor or blender, puree onion-potato mixture and 1 cup milk until smooth. Return to Dutch oven. Add remaining milk, salt, and pepper. Cook until heated through. Makes 4 servings.

Per serving: 188 calories; 9 g protein; 4 g fat; 20% calories from fat; 3 mg cholesterol; 29 g carbohydrates; 557 mg sodium; 3 g fiber

Carrot Soup

4   cups water
2   pounds carrots, peeled and chopped
1½   teaspoons salt, divided
2   tablespoons butter
1   large onion, chopped
2   cloves garlic, minced
1   can (14 fluid ounces) evaporated skim milk
1   tablespoon sugar
1   tablespoon chopped fresh or 1 teaspoon dried dill
½   teaspoon ground allspice
      pepper to taste

In Dutch oven or large saucepan, bring to boil water, carrots, and 1 teaspoon salt. Reduce heat to low; cover and simmer 12 to 15 minutes or until fork-tender. Drain, reserving cooking liquid. Set carrots aside. Heat butter in small skillet over medium heat. Add onion and garlic. Cook until onion is tender, about 5 minutes. In food processor or blender, carefully puree onion mixture and carrots in batches with some reserved cooking liquid until smooth. Return to saucepan. Add milk and enough reserved cooking liquid until desired thickness. Stir in sugar, dill, allspice, and remaining salt and pepper to taste. Cook until heated through. Makes 4 servings.

Per serving: 205 calories; 8 g protein; 5 g fat; 22% calories from fat; 15 mg cholesterol; 33 g carbohydrates; 836 mg sodium; 6 g fiber

Hearty Potato and Greens Soup

2 large potatoes (about 1 1/2 pounds),
    peeled and cut into 1/2-inch pieces
2 cups water
4 ounces fresh greens (escarole, romaine, leaf
    lettuce, etc.), torn (about 4 cups)
1 teaspoon salt
1/2 teaspoon curry powder
1/2 teaspoon ground cumin
1 cup nonfat plain yogurt
1 cup skim milk
2 teaspoons sugar
    lemon wedges for garnish

In Dutch oven or large saucepan, bring to boil potatoes and water. Reduce heat to low; cover and simmer until potatoes are tender, about 7 to 10 minutes. With slotted spoon, remove 1/2 potatoes and put in food processor or blender; let cool slightly. Put remaining half in bowl. Meanwhile, add greens, salt, curry powder, and cumin to saucepan with potato liquid. Cover and cook until greens are tender, about 7 to 15 minutes, depending on greens. Add yogurt to potatoes in food processor; process until smooth. Add potato-yogurt mixture, along with remaining potato, skim milk, and sugar, to green mixture. Heat through over low heat (do not boil or yogurt will curdle). Serve with lemon wedges if desired. Makes 6 servings.

Per serving: 144 calories; 6 g protein; .5 g fat; 2% calories from fat; 1 mg cholesterol; 30 g carbohydrates; 414 mg sodium; 2 g fiber

Beet, Potato, and Celery Salad

$^1/_2$ cup nonfat plain yogurt
$^1/_2$ cup light mayonnaise
2 teaspoons lemon juice
$^1/_2$ teaspoon salt
   pepper to taste
1 can (14.5 ounces) whole beets, drained and cut into
   $^3/_4$-inch pieces
4 medium red potatoes (about 1 pound), cooked and
   cut into $^3/_4$-inch pieces
3 celery ribs, chopped (about 1 $^1/_2$ cups)
1 large dill pickle, chopped (about 1 cup)
   chopped parsley for garnish

In large bowl stir together yogurt, mayonnaise, lemon juice, salt, and pepper. Add beets, potatoes, celery, and pickle; toss until well coated. Cover and refrigerate several hours or overnight. Garnish with parsley, if desired. Makes 6 servings.

Per serving: 175 calories; 3 g protein; 7 g fat; 35% calories from fat; 7 mg cholesterol; 25 g carbohydrates; 744 mg sodium; 3 g fiber

Citrus Soufflé Salad

1   package (4-serving size) lemon-flavored gelatin
1   cup boiling water
1/2 cup cold water
1   tablespoon lemon juice
1/2 cup light mayonnaise
1/4 teaspoon salt
    pepper to taste
3/4 cup low-fat cottage cheese
1/2 cup diced grapefruit sections
1/2 cup diced orange sections
1/2 cup shredded carrot
    greens for garnish

In medium bowl, stir lemon-flavored gelatin and boiling water until gelatin is dissolved. Add cold water, lemon juice, mayonnaise, salt, and pepper until well blended. Pour into 8-inch square metal baking dish; freeze about 15 to 20 minutes or until firm about 1-inch from edge but soft in center. Transfer to large mixing bowl. Beat with mixer until fluffy. Fold in cottage cheese, grapefruit sections, orange sections, and carrot. Pour into 4-cup mold or four individual 1-cup molds. Chill until firm. Serve over greens, if desired. Makes 4 servings.

Per serving: 251 calories; 8 g protein; 11 g fat; 37% calories from fat; 15 mg cholesterol; 32 g carbohydrates; 574 mg sodium; 1 g fiber

Apple and Red Cabbage Slaw

3 medium apples, cored and coarsely shredded
1/2 head (about 1 pound) red cabbage, shredded
4 medium celery ribs, coarsely chopped
1/4 cup raisins
2 tablespoons olive oil
1 tablespoon honey
1 tablespoon lemon juice
  lettuce leaves for garnish

In large bowl, combine apples, cabbage, celery, and raisins. In measuring cup, mix together oil, honey, and lemon juice until well blended. Add to slaw; toss until well coated. Serve on bed of lettuce, if desired. Makes 6 servings.

Per serving: 146 calories; 1 g protein; 5 g fat; 29% calories from fat; 0 mg cholesterol; 27 g carbohydrates; 29 mg sodium; 4 g fiber

Breads and Muffins

Vanilla French Toast

2 cups skim milk
  cholesterol-free, fat-free egg substitute,
    equivalent to 4 eggs
1 tablespoon sugar
2 teaspoons ground cinnamon (optional)
1 teaspoon vanilla extract
8 slices high-fiber multigrain or whole wheat bread

In large baking dish, beat milk, egg substitute, sugar, cinnamon, and vanilla until well blended. Add bread in single layer; cover and refrigerate several hours or overnight, turning once. Spray large nonstick skillet with nonstick cooking spray; place over medium heat. With metal spatula transfer 3-4 slices of egg-soaked bread to skillet. Cook 8 to 12 minutes or until brown and crisp on both sides, turning once. Remove and keep warm. Repeat with remaining slices. Makes 4 servings.

Per 2-slice serving: 193 calories; 10 g protein; 2 g fat; 10% calories from fat; 2 mg cholesterol; 33 g carbohydrates; 300 mg sodium; 3 g fiber

Hearty Cran-Apple Muffins

1   cup all-purpose flour
1/2   cup whole wheat flour or oat bran
3/4   cup firmly packed dark brown sugar
1   teaspoon baking soda
1   teaspoon ground cinnamon
1/4   teaspoon salt
      cholesterol-free, fat-free egg substitute,
        equivalent to 2 eggs
1/4   cup canola, corn, safflower, or sunflower oil
1   teaspoon vanilla extract
3/4   cup diced, unpeeled tart apple
3/4   cup fresh or frozen cranberries

Preheat oven to 350°F. Grease well 6 (2½-inch) muffin cups or line with paper baking cups. In large bowl, mix flours, brown sugar, baking soda, cinnamon, and salt. In separate bowl, blend egg substitute, oil, and vanilla. Add to flour mixture all at once, stirring just until dry ingredients are moistened. Gently stir in apple and cranberries. Spoon into prepared cups. Bake 20 to 25 minutes or until muffins are browned and firm to touch. Makes 6 muffins.

Per muffin: 241 calories; 4 g protein; 7 g fat; 26% calories from fat; 0 mg cholesterol; 41 g carbohydrates; 137 mg sodium; 2 g fiber

Banana-Blueberry Oat Bread

1 1/2 cups old-fashioned rolled oats
1   cup all-purpose flour
1   teaspoon baking powder
1/2   teaspoon baking soda
1/2   teaspoon salt
1   cup sugar
1/3   cup canola, corn, safflower, or sunflower oil
      cholesterol-free, fat-free egg substitute,
          equivalent to 2 eggs
3   tablespoons buttermilk or plain nonfat yogurt
1   cup mashed ripe bananas (about 2)
1/2   cup fresh or frozen blueberries

Preheat oven to 350°F. Grease 9x5-inch loaf pan. Cut 18x5-inch strip waxed paper or foil; place in prepared pan, covering short sides and bottom; set aside. In food processor or blender, process oats until consistency of flour. In large bowl, mix processed oats, flour, baking powder, baking soda, and salt. In separate bowl, blend sugar, oil, egg substitute, buttermilk or yogurt, and bananas. Add to flour mixture, stirring until well blended. Stir in blueberries. Spoon into prepared pan. Bake 50 to 60 minutes or until pick inserted in center comes out clean. Remove from pan to wire rack; cool completely. Makes 1 loaf (16 slices).

Per slice: 78 calories; 3 g protein; .5 g fat; 7% calories from fat; 0 mg cholesterol; 15 g carbohydrates; 128 mg sodium; 1.5 g fiber

Oat and Pumpkin Muffins

1 1/2   cups oat bran
 1/2   cup all-purpose flour
  2   teaspoons baking powder
  1   teaspoon pumpkin pie spice
 1/4   teaspoon salt
  1   cup canned or fresh mashed cooked pumpkin
 2/3   cup firmly packed brown sugar
 1/2   cup skim milk
  2   egg whites
  2   tablespoons canola, corn, safflower, or sunflower oil

Preheat oven to 425°F. Grease well 12 (2 1/2-inch) muffin cups or line with paper baking cups. In large bowl, mix oat bran, flour, baking powder, pumpkin pie spice, and salt. In separate bowl, blend pumpkin, brown sugar, skim milk, egg whites, and oil. Add to oat bran/flour mixture all at once, stirring until dry ingredients are moistened. Spoon into prepared muffin cups. Bake 18 to 20 minutes or until muffins are firm to touch. Makes 12 muffins.

Per muffin: 125 calories; 4 g protein; 3 g fat; 18% calories from fat; 0 mg cholesterol; 26 g carbohydrates; 122 mg sodium; 2 g fiber

Pizza Bagel

2 tablespoons canola, corn, safflower, or sunflower oil
1 medium onion, cut into thin wedges
1 large potato (about 6 to 7 ounces), cooked, peeled, and cut into 1/4-inch slices
1/2 large green pepper, seeded and cut into strips
1 teaspoon dried oregano
1/2 teaspoon salt
2 bagels (oat bran, pumpernickel, or plain), cut in half
1 cup shredded skim-milk mozzarella cheese (4 ounces)

Preheat broiler. Heat oil in large nonstick skillet over medium heat. Add onion, potato, and green pepper. Cook, stirring occasionally, 5 to 8 minutes or until onion is browned. Stir in oregano and salt. Place bagels, cut side up, on broiler pan. Broil until lightly toasted. Top each bagel half with 1/4 onion-potato mixture and sprinkle with 1/4 cheese. Broil until cheese is melted and lightly browned. Makes 4 servings.

Variation: Omit green pepper, oregano, and salt. Cook onion and potato as above. Stir in 1 can (8 ounces) sliced beets, well drained and rinsed. Continue as directed above.

Per serving: 245 calories; 11 g protein; 8 g fat; 32% calories from fat; 16 mg cholesterol; 30 g carbohydrates; 551 mg sodium; 2 g fiber

Apple Gingerbread Scones

1/3 cup skim milk
1/3 cup light molasses
3 tablespoons unsweetened applesauce
2 cups all-purpose flour
2 teaspoons baking powder
1 teaspoon ground cinnamon
1 teaspoon ground ginger
1/4 teaspoon baking soda
1/4 teaspoon ground cloves
4 tablespoons cold butter, cut up

Preheat oven to 425°F. In small bowl or measuring cup, mix milk, molasses, and applesauce; set aside. In large bowl, combine flour, baking powder, cinnamon, ginger, baking soda, and cloves. With pastry blender or fingers cut in butter until mixture resembles fine granules. Pour in milk mixture and stir with fork to form a smooth, soft dough. On lightly floured surface, knead dough 10 to 12 times. Cut dough in half. Knead each half into ball. On ungreased baking sheet, pat each piece into 5-inch circle. Cut into 6 wedges; separate slightly. Bake 10 to 12 minutes or until crusty and hollow-sounding when tapped. Serve warm. Makes 12 scones.

Per scone: 132 calories; 2 g protein; 4 g fat; 28% calories from fat; 10 mg cholesterol; 21 g carbohydrates; 109 mg sodium; trace g fiber

Main Dishes: Poultry and Fish

Jalapeño Turkey Bake

1   cup uncooked long-grain brown rice
3   cups, 3/4-inch cubes, cooked turkey breast
      (about 12 ounces)
1   can (10 ounces) enchilada sauce
2   fresh jalapeño peppers, seeded, chopped
      (about 1/4 cup)
1 1/2   cups frozen or canned (drained) whole kernel corn
1/4   cup chopped green pepper
3/4   teaspoon salt
1   cup nonfat sour cream
      additional chopped jalapeño peppers and chopped
      cilantro for garnish (optional)

Preheat oven to 350°F. Grease shallow 1 1/2-quart casserole or 11x7-inch baking dish. Prepare rice according to package directions. In large bowl stir cooked rice, turkey, enchilada sauce, chopped jalapeño peppers, corn, green pepper, and salt until well blended. Spoon into prepared casserole. Cover and bake 25 to 30 minutes or until heated through. To serve, spoon sour cream over top and sprinkle with jalapeño peppers and cilantro, if desired. Makes 6 servings.

Per serving: 346 calories; 26 g protein; 2 g fat; 7% calories from fat; 55 mg cholesterol; 52 g carbohydrates; 1,083 mg sodium; 3 g fiber

Moroccan-Style Chicken and Couscous

1 whole chicken breast (about 1½ pounds), split, skinned, and cut in half
1 medium onion, sliced
2 medium carrots, cut into 1-inch pieces
1 teaspoon turmeric
1 teaspoon salt
¼ teaspoon pepper
2 cups cooked chickpeas
2 medium zucchini, cut into ½-inch pieces
2 cups shredded cabbage (about 4 ounces)
1 large tomato, chopped
2 tablespoons chopped parsley
2 tablespoons chopped cilantro
1 package (10 ounces) plain couscous

In Dutch oven or large saucepan, bring to boil 3 cups water, chicken, onion, carrots, turmeric, salt, and pepper. Reduce heat to medium-low; cover and cook 30 minutes. Add chickpeas, zucchini, cabbage, tomato, parsley, and cilantro. Cover and cook 15 to 20 minutes more or until chicken and vegetables are fork-tender. Meanwhile, prepare couscous according to package directions. To serve, place ¼ couscous in shallow bowl; top with ¼ chicken-broth mixture. Makes 4 servings.

Per serving: 382 calories; 29 g protein; 4 g fat; 11% calories from fat; 43 mg cholesterol; 57 g carbohydrates; 415 mg sodium; 6 g fiber

Turkey Tabbouleh

1 1/2 cups warm water
1 cup uncooked bulgar
2 tablespoons olive oil
3 cups coarsely chopped, cooked turkey breast
   (about 12 ounces)
3 green onions with tops, sliced
1 large Granny Smith or Winesap apple, cored
   and chopped
1 celery rib, finely chopped
1 clove garlic, minced
1/2 cup finely chopped parsley
1/4 cup finely chopped red onion
1 cup nonfat plain yogurt
1/2 teaspoon salt
   pepper to taste
2 tablespoons sliced almonds for garnish

In large bowl, place water, bulgar, and olive oil; let stand at least 30 minutes or until all liquid has been absorbed. Add chopped turkey, green onions, apple, celery, garlic, parsley, red onion, yogurt, salt, and pepper; toss to combine. Chill at least 30 minutes to blend flavors. To serve, sprinkle with almonds, if desired. Makes 8 servings.

Per serving: 227 calories; 20 g protein; 6 g fat; 25% calories from fat; 37 mg cholesterol; 22 g carbohydrates; 196 mg sodium; 5 g fiber

Summer Chicken Salad

3   cups, $3/4$-inch cubes, cooked chicken breast
     (about 12 ounces)
3   cups $3/4$-inch melon balls or cubes (cantaloupe,
     honeydew, cassava, etc.)
1   large celery rib, chopped
$1/3$ cup light mayonnaise
$1/4$ cup chopped walnuts
$1/2$ teaspoon salt
     lettuce leaves for garnish

In large bowl place chicken cubes, melon, celery, mayonnaise, walnuts, and salt; toss until well blended. Serve over lettuce, if desired. Makes 4 servings.

Variation: If desired, omit melon balls and substitute 3 cups fresh or drained canned peach slices.

Per serving: 273 calories; 24 g protein; 14 g fat; 46% calories from fat; 65 mg cholesterol; 13 g carbohydrates; 478 mg sodium; 2 g fiber

Chicken and Rice Cajun-Style

2 cups, 3/4-inch cubes, cooked chicken or turkey breast (about 8 ounces)
1 cup cooked brown rice
1 can (16 ounces) stewed tomatoes, undrained
1 medium onion, chopped (about 1/2 cup)
1 medium celery rib, finely chopped
1/2 cup finely chopped green or red pepper
1 small yellow squash, cut into 1/2-inch cubes
1 clove garlic, minced
1/4 teaspoon dried thyme
1/4 teaspoon crushed hot red pepper, or to taste
1/4 teaspoon ground cloves
1/4 teaspoon ground allspice
1/3 cup Italian seasoned bread crumbs

Preheat oven to 350°F. Place all ingredients except bread crumbs in lightly greased 2-quart casserole. Stir until well blended. Top evenly with bread crumbs. Bake 35 to 40 minutes or until heated through. Makes 4 servings.

Per serving: 253 calories; 25 g protein; 4 g fat; 15% calories from fat; 59 mg cholesterol; 27 g carbohydrates; 304 mg sodium; 3 g fiber

Asparagus, Mushroom, and Chicken Stir-Fry

1   tablespoon cornstarch
1   tablespoon chicken bouillon granules
3   tablespoons soy sauce
1   cup water, divided
4   tablespoons canola, corn, safflower, or
      sunflower oil, divided
12 ounces boneless, skinless chicken breast, cut into
      2x1-inch strips
1   pound fresh asparagus, cut diagonally into
      2-inch pieces
4   ounces fresh mushrooms, sliced
6   green onions, cut into 1-inch pieces
½   cup sliced canned water chestnuts
1½ cups halved cherry tomatoes
      cooked brown rice (optional)

In small bowl or measuring cup, stir cornstarch, bouillon granules, and soy sauce into ¾ cup water until well blended; set aside. Heat 2 tablespoons oil in large skillet or wok over medium-high heat. Add chicken; cook, stirring constantly, 2 minutes or until chicken is white. Remove chicken; keep warm. Add 1 tablespoon oil to skillet. Add asparagus. Stir to coat with oil. Add remaining ¼ cup water; cover and cook 3 minutes. Remove cover; add remaining tablespoon oil, mushrooms, green onions, and water chestnuts. Cook, stirring constantly, 4 minutes or until asparagus is tender-crisp.

Add reserved chicken and tomatoes and then cornstarch mixture. Cook, gently stirring constantly, 2 minutes or until sauce thickens, bubbles, and tomatoes are heated through. Serve over hot cooked brown rice, if desired. Makes 4 servings.

Per serving: 245 calories; 25 g protein; 10 g fat; 37% calories from fat; 54 mg cholesterol; 14 g carbohydrates; 1,109 mg sodium; 4 g fiber

Chicken and Peanut Stir-Fry

2 whole chicken breasts, split, boned, skinned, and cut into bite-size pieces
1/2 cup dry sherry
1/2 teaspoon minced fresh ginger
2 tablespoons canola, corn, safflower, or sunflower oil
1 medium onion, chopped
1 small carrot, cut diagonally into thin slices
1 medium green pepper, cut into strips
1/2 cup sliced fresh mushrooms
1/2 cup broccoli florets
1/4 cup unsalted dry-roasted peanuts
1/2 teaspoon salt
   pepper to taste
2 cups hot, cooked brown rice

In small bowl, toss chicken, sherry, and ginger; let stand 2 hours to marinate. Heat oil in large skillet or wok over medium-high heat. Add onion; cook, stirring constantly, 2 minutes or until onion is tender-crisp. Remove chicken from marinade, reserving marinade, and place in skillet or wok. Cook, stirring constantly, 5 minutes or until chicken turns white. Add carrots and green pepper; cook, stirring constantly, 3 minutes. Add mushroom, broccoli, and peanuts. Add reserved marinade, salt, and pepper. Cook, stirring constantly, 1 to 2 minutes or until sauce thickens and vegetables are tender-crisp. Serve over hot cooked brown rice. Makes 4 servings.

Per serving: 492 calories; 40 g protein; 16 g fat; 31% calories from fat; 95 mg cholesterol; 35 g carbohydrates; 369 mg sodium; 3 g fiber

All-in-One Fish Dinner

1 pound boneless, skinless, fresh or frozen (thawed) fish fillets (cod, haddock, or pollack), cut into serving pieces
1/2 teaspoon salt
pepper to taste
1 tablespoon canola, corn, safflower, or sunflower oil
1 large onion, thinly sliced
1 small clove garlic, minced
1 can (8 ounces) tomato sauce
1 cup hot water
1/4 teaspoon dried fennel or dill
dash cayenne pepper
2 medium potatoes, peeled and thinly sliced
1/2 cup frozen or canned (drained) peas

Preheat oven to 350°F. Grease 2½-quart shallow casserole or baking dish. Sprinkle fish with salt and pepper. Heat oil in medium skillet over medium heat. Add onion and garlic; cook 5 minutes or until onion is tender. Stir in tomato sauce, water, fennel, and cayenne pepper. In prepared casserole, layer fish, potatoes, and peas, ending with potatoes. Pour tomato-onion sauce over fish and vegetables. Cover and bake 40 minutes. Remove cover and cook 10 to 15 minutes longer or until fish flakes easily when tested with fork. Makes 4 servings.

Per serving: 245 calories; 24 g protein; 4 g fat; 17% calories from fat; 48 mg cholesterol; 27 g carbohydrates; 676 mg sodium; 4 g fiber

Sesame-Ginger Haddock

1 pound boneless, skinless, fresh or frozen (thawed),
   haddock fillets
1/2 teaspoon salt
1 1/2 tablespoons butter
2 tablespoons minced green onion with tops
2 tablespoons toasted sesame seeds
1/2 teaspoon grated fresh or 1/4 teaspoon ground ginger

Preheat oven to 350°F. Grease shallow 2 1/2-quart casserole or baking dish. Sprinkle fish with salt; place in single layer in casserole. Melt butter in small skillet over low heat. Add green onion, sesame seeds, and ginger; cook 2 minutes. Spoon evenly over fish. Bake 15 to 25 minutes or until fish flakes easily when tested with fork. Makes 4 servings.

Per serving: 165 calories; 24 g protein; 7 g fat; 41% calories from fat; 74 mg cholesterol; trace g carbohydrates; 379 mg sodium; 0 g fiber

Flounder with Fresh Orange Sauce

1   pound boneless, skinless, fresh or frozen (thawed)
     flounder fillets
1/2 teaspoon salt
     pepper to taste
1/4 teaspoon ground ginger
1/2 cup orange juice
2   tablespoons lemon juice
1   green onion with top, thinly sliced
1   medium tomato, peeled and chopped
1/4 medium green pepper, chopped
1   tablespoon butter, melted
3   oranges, peeled and thinly sliced

Preheat oven to 350°F. Grease 2¹/2-quart shallow casserole or baking dish. Sprinkle fish with mixture of salt, pepper, and ginger and place in shallow dish or bowl. Add orange and lemon juice to fish; let stand 20 minutes. Lightly drain fish, reserving remaining marinade; place in prepared casserole. Top with green onion, tomato, and green pepper. Drizzle evenly with butter. Bake 10 minutes. Pour reserved marinade over fish; top with orange slices. Bake 15 minutes more or until fish flakes easily when tested with fork. Makes 4 servings.

Per serving: 199 calories; 23 g protein; 4 g fat; 20% calories from fat; 62 mg cholesterol; 17 g carbohydrates; 386 mg sodium; 3 g fiber

Onion-Dill Halibut

4   halibut steaks (4 ounces each), fresh or
    frozen (thawed)
1/2 teaspoon salt
    pepper to taste
2   large onions, thinly sliced
1   tablespoon butter
1   tablespoon olive oil
1   tablespoon fresh chopped or 1 teaspoon dried dill

Preheat oven to 400°F. Season halibut steaks evenly with salt
and pepper. In 9-inch square baking dish, place onions, butter,
oil, and dill. Bake 10 to 15 minutes or until onions begin to
brown. Remove 1/4 onions; place steaks in baking dish and top
with reserved onions. Bake 10 to 15 minutes or until fish flakes
easily when tested with fork. Makes 4 servings.

Per serving: 176 calories; 18 g protein; 8 g fat; 44%
calories from fat; 35 mg cholesterol; 6 g carbohydrates;
338 mg sodium; 1 g fiber

Easy Turkey Lasagna

9 lasagna noodles
1 pound raw, ground white meat turkey
1 small onion, chopped
1 jar (28 ounces) spaghetti sauce with mushrooms
   (or your favorite sauce)
1 cup part-skim ricotta cheese
2 tablespoons chopped parsley
2 tablespoons grated Parmesan cheese
2 tablespoons skim milk
1/8 teaspoon ground pepper
3 ounces part-skim-milk mozzarella cheese,
   shredded (3/4 cup)

Preheat oven to 350°F. Grease 11x7-inch baking dish; set aside. Cook lasagna noodles according to package directions; drain and rinse. Meanwhile, in medium nonstick skillet over medium-high heat, cook ground turkey and onion until turkey is brown. Drain off fat. Remove from heat; stir in spaghetti sauce. In small bowl, mix together ricotta cheese, parsley, Parmesan cheese, milk, and pepper. In prepared dish, arrange 3 lasagna noodles in single layer; top with 2/3 turkey-sauce mixture, then with 1/2 cheese mixture; repeat. Top with remaining noodles, remaining turkey-sauce mixture, then mozzarella. Bake 40 to 50 minutes or until bubbly and heated through. Let stand 5 minutes before serving. Makes 8 servings.

Per serving: 355 calories; 24 g protein; 12 g fat; 30% calories from fat; 71 mg cholesterol; 37 g carbohydrates; 635 mg sodium; 3 g fiber

Main Dishes: Vegetarian

Spinach-Garlic Fettuccine

8 ounces uncooked fettuccine
3 tablespoons olive oil
3 large cloves garlic, minced
3/4 pound fresh spinach, trimmed, washed, and torn
   into bite-size pieces (about 8 cups)
1/3 cup grated Parmesan cheese
1/2 teaspoon salt
   pepper to taste
   dash ground nutmeg

Cook fettuccine according to package directions. Meanwhile, heat oil in Dutch oven or 12-inch skillet over medium heat. Add garlic; cook 2 to 3 minutes or until lightly brown. Add spinach; cook, stirring occasionally, 5 minutes or until spinach is limp and tender. Drain fettuccine. In large serving bowl, toss fettuccine, spinach mixture, cheese, salt, pepper, and nutmeg until well blended. Serve immediately. Makes 4 servings.

Per serving: 305 calories; 10 g protein; 12 g fat; 37% calories from fat; 5 mg cholesterol; 38 g carbohydrates; 448 mg sodium; 5 g fiber

Green Vegetable Spaghetti Sauce

2   tablespoons canola, corn, safflower, or sunflower oil
2   green onions with tops, sliced
1   clove garlic, minced
1   cup vegetable broth, divided
3   medium tomatoes, chopped
1   package (10 ounces) fresh or frozen (thawed)
       Brussels sprouts, cut into quarters
10 ounces fresh or 1 package (9 ounces) frozen
       (thawed) whole green beans, cut into 1-inch pieces
1   teaspoon dried basil
1   teaspoon dried oregano
1/2 teaspoon salt
     pepper to taste
2   teaspoons cornstarch
1/4 cup fresh or frozen peas
1/4 cup chopped fresh or 2 tablespoons dried parsley
6   ounces spaghetti, cooked and hot

Heat oil in large skillet over medium heat. Add green onions and garlic; cook 1 minute. Add 1/2 cup broth, tomatoes, Brussels sprouts, green beans, basil, oregano, salt, and pepper. Cook, covered, about 8 to 12 minutes or until Brussels sprouts are tender. Stir cornstarch into remaining 1/2 cup broth. Add to skillet with peas and parsley. Cook, stirring occasionally, until thickened and vegetables are tender. Serve over hot spaghetti. Makes 4 servings.

Per serving: 275 calories; 9 g protein; 8 g fat; 24% calories from fat; 0 mg cholesterol; 45 g carbohydrates; 307 mg sodium; 8 g fiber

Tomato-Onion Stuffed Eggplant

2   small eggplants (about 3/4 pound each)
1   tablespoon olive oil
1   tablespoon butter
2   medium onions, thinly sliced
2   cloves garlic, minced
3   medium tomatoes (about 1 pound), peeled,
     seeded, and chopped
1/2 cup finely chopped fresh parsley
1/2 teaspoon salt
1   bay leaf
1   stick (2 inches) cinnamon
     pepper to taste
8   black olives, coarsely chopped

Grease shallow 2½-quart baking dish. Cut top stem and cap from eggplant. Heat oil in large nonstick skillet over medium-high heat. Add eggplants; cook 5 minutes, or until tender, turning often. Cut in half lengthwise; scoop out pulp, leaving thin shell. Coarsely chop pulp. Set eggplant shells and pulp aside. Heat butter in same skillet over medium heat; add onions and garlic. Cook 5 to 8 minutes or until golden brown. Add tomatoes and reserved eggplant pulp; cook 10 minutes. Preheat oven to 375°F. Add parsley, salt, bay leaf, cinnamon stick, and pepper to skillet; cook 10 minutes. Remove bay leaf and cinnamon stick. Place reserved eggplant shells in prepared baking dish. Place ¼ tomato-eggplant mixture into each. Top with chopped olives. Bake 10 minutes or until heated through. Makes 4 servings.

Per serving: 165 calories; 4 g protein; 9 g fat; 44% calories from fat; 7 mg cholesterol; 22 g carbohydrates; 381 mg sodium; 9 g fiber

Sesame Vegetable Stir-Fry

1   tablespoon canola, corn, safflower, or sunflower oil
1   small clove garlic, finely minced
1   teaspoon finely minced fresh or ½ teaspoon
     ground ginger
3/4 pound broccoli, trimmed and cut into florets
3   medium carrots, peeled and thinly sliced
3   medium leeks (white part only), thinly sliced
2   tablespoons vegetable broth
1   tablespoon toasted sesame seeds
1   teaspoon soy sauce
1   teaspoon Oriental sesame oil

Heat oil in large skillet or wok over medium-high heat. Add garlic and ginger; cook, stirring constantly, 15 seconds. Reduce heat to medium. Add broccoli, carrots, and leeks; cook, stirring constantly, 1 minute. Add broth; cover and cook 3 minutes. Increase heat to high; uncover and cook, stirring constantly, 5 minutes or until vegetables are tender. Add sesame seeds, soy sauce, and sesame oil; toss until well coated. Serve immediately. Makes 4 servings.

Per serving: 123 calories; 3 g protein; 6 g fat; 41% calories from fat; 0 mg cholesterol; 16 g carbohydrates; 131 mg sodium; 5 g fiber

Red Beans and Rice

2   tablespoons olive oil
1   medium onion, chopped
1-2   cloves garlic, minced
1   large celery rib with leaves, thinly sliced
½   cup chopped green pepper
4   cups water or vegetable broth
1   cup uncooked long-grain brown rice
1   teaspoon salt
½   teaspoon dried thyme
    crushed red pepper or liquid hot pepper sauce to taste
2   cans (15½ to 19 ounces) red kidney beans, rinsed
    and drained

Heat oil in Dutch oven or large saucepan over medium heat. Add onion, garlic, celery, and green pepper. Cook 5 minutes or until vegetables are tender. Add water, rice, salt, thyme, and red pepper to taste. Bring to boil over high heat. Reduce heat to simmer; cover and cook 40 to 45 minutes or until rice is almost tender. Stir in beans; cover and cook until beans are heated through and rice is tender. Makes 5 servings.

Per serving: 357 calories; 14 g protein; 6 g fat; 16% calories from fat; 0 mg cholesterol; 62 g carbohydrates; 439 mg sodium; 12 g fiber

Zucchini and Rice Casserole

1	tablespoon canola, corn, safflower, or sunflower oil
1	cup uncooked brown rice
1	teaspoon grated fresh ginger
3	green onions with tops, chopped
3	medium zucchini, sliced
1/2	medium green pepper, seeded and chopped
3	small tomatoes, cored and cut into eighths
2³/4	cups boiling vegetable broth
1	teaspoon soy sauce
1	clove garlic, minced

Preheat oven to 350°F. Grease shallow 2¹/2-quart casserole. Heat oil in large skillet over medium-low heat. Add rice and ginger; cook, stirring, 5 minutes or until rice is golden brown. Spoon evenly into prepared casserole; top with layers of green onion, zucchini, green pepper, and tomato. Stir together broth, soy sauce, and garlic; pour over vegetable-rice mixture. Cover and bake 1 hour and 15 minutes or until rice and vegetables are tender. Makes 6 servings.

Per serving: 151 calories; 3 g protein; 3 g fat; 18% calories from fat; 0 mg cholesterol; 28 g carbohydrates; 64 mg sodium; 2 g fiber

Barbecued Bean Casserole

2 tablespoons canola, corn, safflower, or sunflower oil
1 small onion, chopped
1 clove garlic, minced
1 can (16 ounces) vegetarian baked beans
1 package (10 ounces) frozen or 1 can (15½ ounces) drained lima beans (about 2 cups)
1 can (15½ to 19 ounces) or 2 cups cooked red kidney beans, rinsed and drained
½ cup catsup
3 tablespoons apple cider vinegar
1 tablespoon brown sugar
1 teaspoon salt
1 teaspoon dry mustard
¼ teaspoon pepper

Preheat oven to 350°F. Heat oil in heat-and-oven-proof 2-quart casserole over medium-high heat. Add onion and garlic; cook 5 minutes or until onion is tender. Stir in remaining ingredients. Bake 45 minutes or until heated through and bubbly. Makes 6 servings.

Per serving: 266 calories; 12 g protein; 6 g fat; 19% calories from fat; 4 mg cholesterol; 44 g carbohydrates; 911 mg sodium; 13 g fiber

Veggie Pockets

3/4 cup low-fat cottage cheese
1/4 cup crumbled blue cheese
1   tablespoon tarragon or apple cider vinegar
1/4 teaspoon dried Italian herb seasoning
1/2 large cucumber, cut in half lengthwise and then
     sliced (about 1/2 cup)
1   medium tomato, diced
1   medium carrot, peeled and shredded
1/2 cup broccoli florets, cut into bite-size pieces
1/4 cup shelled sunflower seeds
4   (6-inch) whole wheat or plain pita breads, cut in half
     alfalfa sprouts for garnish

In large bowl, gently mix cottage cheese, blue cheese, vinegar, and seasoning until well blended. Add cucumber, tomato, carrot, broccoli, and sunflower seeds; toss until well blended. Spoon 1/8 vegetable-cheese mixture into each pita half. Top with alfalfa sprouts, if desired. Makes 4 servings.

Per serving: 295 calories; 16 g protein; 8 g fat; 24% calories from fat; 11 mg cholesterol; 41 g carbohydrates; 595 mg sodium; 3 g fiber

Vegetable Side Dishes

Pineapple and Yam Casserole

2   pounds fresh yams (about 2 large), peeled and cut into 1-inch pieces
1   cup water
1   cup unsweetened pineapple juice
2   tablespoons lemon juice
2   teaspoons cornstarch
1   teaspoon sugar
¼   teaspoon salt
½   fresh pineapple (about 3½ pounds), peeled, cored, and cut into 1-inch pieces
1   green onion with top, sliced
1   small celery rib, diagonally sliced (¼ cup)

In Dutch oven or large saucepan, over medium heat, cook yams in water, covered, about 10 to 15 minutes or until almost tender. Drain. In same Dutch oven, over medium heat, cook, stirring constantly, pineapple juice, lemon juice, cornstarch, sugar, and salt until thickened and bubbly. Add drained yams, pineapple pieces, green onions, and celery. Reduce heat to low; cover and cook until heated through, about 5 minutes. Makes 6 servings.

Per serving: 216 calories; 3 g protein; .5 g fat; 2% calories from fat; 0 mg cholesterol; 51 g carbohydrates; 112 mg sodium; 5 g fiber

Yam Soufflé

1   cup mashed yams—fresh cooked, canned, or
       frozen (thawed)
1/2   cup firmly packed brown sugar
1/4   teaspoon ground nutmeg
1/2   teaspoon grated orange peel
1/8   teaspoon salt
3   egg whites, at room temperature
1/8   teaspoon cream of tartar

Preheat oven to 350°F. Grease 1-quart casserole or baking dish. In medium bowl, stir yams, brown sugar, nutmeg, orange peel, and salt until well blended. In small bowl, beat egg whites and cream of tartar with mixer at high speed until stiff peaks form. Gently fold into yam mixture and then spoon into prepared casserole. Place in pan of hot water. Bake 35 to 40 minutes or until puffed and starts to pull away from sides. Makes 4 servings.

Per serving: 173 calories; 3 g protein; .5 g fat; 1% calories from fat; 0 mg cholesterol; 40 g carbohydrates; 350 mg sodium; 1 g fiber

Garlicky Black Bean Dip

2 cans (15 ounces each) black beans, drained
1 medium onion, coarsely chopped
1 small green pepper, coarsely chopped
2 cloves garlic, chopped
3 tablespoons red wine vinegar
3 tablespoons olive oil
1 teaspoon sugar
1 teaspoon salt
   pepper to taste
   baked tortilla chips and/or raw vegetable dippers

In food processor or blender, place beans, onion, green pepper, garlic, vinegar, oil, sugar, salt, and pepper. Process until beans are coarsely mashed or of desired consistency. Serve with chips and/or vegetables, if desired. Makes 4 cups, 32 servings (2 tablespoons).

Per serving: 37 calories; 1 g protein; 1 g fat; 32% calories from fat; 0 mg cholesterol; 4 g carbohydrates; 67 mg sodium; 2 g fiber

Asparagus-Cheese Casserole

1½ pounds fresh or 2 packages (10 ounces each) frozen
    asparagus, cooked
2   tablespoons canola, corn, safflower, or sunflower oil
1   medium onion, chopped
1   clove garlic, minced
1   can (16 ounces) tomatoes, undrained
1   teaspoon salt
¼   teaspoon dried thyme
¼   teaspoon liquid hot pepper sauce
1   can (8 ounces) tomato sauce
4   ounces part-skim-milk mozzarella, shredded
2   tablespoons grated Parmesan cheese

Preheat oven to 350°F. In shallow baking pan or casserole,
arrange asparagus; set aside. Heat oil in medium saucepan over
medium heat. Add onion and garlic; cook 5 minutes or until
lightly browned. Add tomatoes, salt, thyme, and pepper sauce.
Reduce heat to low. Cook, uncovered, 20 minutes. Add tomato sauce. Cook 20 minutes or until flavors blend. Pour sauce
evenly over asparagus; top with cheeses. Bake 20 to 25 minutes
or until asparagus is heated and cheese melts. Makes 8 servings.

Per serving: 119 calories; 7 g protein; 6 g fat; 47% calories
from fat; 8 mg cholesterol; 9 g carbohydrates; 630 mg
sodium; 2 g fiber

Green Bean and Olive Toss

1   package (9 ounces) frozen French-cut green beans
¼   cup sliced pitted black olives
1   tablespoon olive oil
1   tablespoon red wine vinegar
¼   teaspoon salt
¼   teaspoon crushed dried oregano
⅛   teaspoon garlic powder
     pepper to taste

Cook green beans according to package directions. In the meantime, in small saucepan over medium heat, cook olives, oil, vinegar, salt, oregano, garlic powder, and pepper until heated through (about 3-5 minutes). Drain green beans; place on serving platter. Pour olive mixture over beans; toss well. Serve immediately. Makes 4 servings.

Per serving: 59 calories; 1 g protein; 5 g fat; 68% calories from fat; 4 mg cholesterol; 0 g carbohydrates; 195 mg sodium; 2 g fiber

Asian-Style Green Beans

2   tablespoons peanut oil
1   small onion, finely chopped
1   clove garlic, minced
2   tablespoons shredded lemon peel
$\frac{1}{2}$ teaspoon dried chili pepper
1   pound fresh trimmed, or 2 packages (9 ounces each) frozen (thawed), whole green beans
1   teaspoon salt
   pinch sugar

Heat oil in large skillet over medium heat. Add onion, garlic, lemon peel, and chili pepper. Cook, stirring constantly, 3 minutes. Reduce heat to low. Add green beans; toss to coat well. Cover and cook 5 minutes or until barely tender, adding water, if necessary. Makes 6 servings.

Per serving: 73 calories; 2 g protein; 4 g fat; 52% calories from fat; 0 mg cholesterol; 8 g carbohydrates; 360 mg sodium; 2 g fiber

Asparagus Vinaigrette

1   teaspoon dill weed, divided
    water
40 thin (1/2-inch thick) asparagus, trimmed and washed
3   tablespoons olive oil
1   teaspoon salt
1/2 teaspoon dry mustard
1/2 teaspoon cracked pepper
3   tablespoons tarragon white-wine vinegar
    lemon wedges for garnish

In large skillet over medium heat, bring 1/2 teaspoon dill weed and 2 inches water to boil. Add asparagus; cook 3 minutes or until fork-tender. Remove; run under cold water. Drain well. To make vinaigrette dressing: In small bowl, stir remaining 1/2 teaspoon dill weed, oil, salt, mustard, and pepper until well blended. Add vinegar; stir until well blended. To serve: Toss asparagus with enough dressing to coat lightly. Serve with additional dressing and lemon wedges, if desired. Makes 4 servings.

Note: If desired, use a smaller number of thicker asparagus. Cook 2 to 3 minutes longer. Proceed as directed above.

Per serving: 88 calories; 3 g protein; 7 g fat; 66% calories from fat; 0 mg cholesterol; 5 g carbohydrates; 182 mg sodium; 2 g fiber

Skewered Brussels Sprouts

1   container (10 ounces) fresh Brussels sprouts, trimmed
     water
1¹/2 tablespoons butter, melted
1¹/2 tablespoons lemon juice
     paprika to taste
     pepper to taste

Preheat grill or broiler. In medium skillet over medium-high heat, cook Brussels sprouts in 1 inch boiling water for 7 to 10 minutes or until tender-crisp. Drain. In medium bowl, mix butter and lemon juice. Add Brussels sprouts; toss to coat well. Thread coated Brussels sprouts on skewers. Sprinkle with paprika and pepper. Grill or broil 2 to 3 minutes or until brown, turning once. Makes 4 servings.

Per serving: 66 calories; 2 g protein; 4 g fat; 53% calories from fat; 11 mg cholesterol; 6 g carbohydrates; 44 mg sodium; 3 g fiber

Lemon Dill Beets

8   medium whole fresh beets, scrubbed well
      with tops removed
1   tablespoon butter
1   tablespoon lemon juice
1¹/₂ teaspoons chopped fresh dill

Preheat grill or broiler. Place beets in center of large piece of heavy-duty foil; fold edges up around beets. Add butter, lemon juice, and dill. Seal edges of foil tightly. Place over grill. Cook, turning frequently, 45 minutes or until beets are tender. Makes 4 servings.

Per serving: 57 calories; 1 g protein; 3 g fat; 45% calories from fat; 7 mg cholesterol; 7 g carbohydrates; 73 mg sodium; 2 g fiber

Lemon Broccoli

1   tablespoon cornstarch
1/4 teaspoon salt
1/4 teaspoon pepper
1   cup skim milk
2   tablespoons lemon juice
1   tablespoon butter
1   tablespoon chopped parsley
1   large head broccoli, trimmed, or 2 packages
      (10 ounces each) frozen broccoli spears,
      cooked and drained

In 1-quart saucepan, mix cornstarch, salt, and pepper. Gradually stir in milk until smooth. Place over medium heat. Bring to boil, stirring constantly. Boil 1 minute. Remove from heat; stir in lemon juice, butter, and parsley. In shallow serving dish, arrange hot broccoli; top with hot lemon sauce. Makes 8 servings.

Per serving: 48 calories; 3 g protein; 2 g fat; 27% calories from fat; 4 mg cholesterol; 6 g carbohydrates; 112 mg sodium; 2 g fiber

Creamy Broccoli-Rice Casserole

2   tablespoons butter
1   medium onion, chopped
1   package (10 ounces) frozen chopped broccoli, thawed
1   can (10 1/2 ounces) cream of chicken soup
1/4   teaspoon garlic salt
1/4   teaspoon celery salt
1/4   teaspoon onion salt
2   cups hot cooked brown rice
1   ounce Swiss cheese, shredded (1/4 cup)

Preheat oven to 350°F. Grease 1 1/2-quart casserole. Heat butter in medium nonstick skillet over medium heat. Add onion; cook 5 minutes or until tender. Add broccoli; cook 3 minutes. Add undiluted soup, garlic, celery, and onion salt. Cook until bubbly, stirring occasionally. Pack rice in greased 2-cup mold or small bowl; invert into center of prepared casserole. Pour broccoli mixture around rice. Sprinkle with cheese. Bake 10 minutes or until cheese melts. Makes 4 servings.

Per serving: 270 calories; 9 g protein; 10 g fat; 33% calories from fat; 20 mg cholesterol; 37 g carbohydrates; 645 mg sodium; 4 g fiber

Tex-Mex Potatoes

1½ cups water
4 medium potatoes (about 1½ pounds), peeled and
cut into ¼-inch-thick slices
½ teaspoon salt
3 tablespoons canola, corn, safflower, or sunflower oil
4 green onions with tops, thinly sliced (½ cup)
1 can (4 ounces) diced green chilies, drained
1 medium clove garlic, minced
4 ounces Monterey Jack cheese, shredded (1 cup)
finely chopped cilantro for garnish

In 10-inch skillet over high heat, bring water to boil. Add potatoes and salt. Reduce heat to medium. Cook, covered, 10 to 12 minutes or until tender; drain.

In same, well-dried, skillet, heat oil over medium heat. Add green onions, chilies, and garlic. Cook, stirring often, 2 minutes. Add potatoes; toss to mix well. Cook 5 to 10 minutes or until potatoes begin to brown, occasionally stirring gently. Sprinkle top with cheese. Reduce heat to low. Cook until cheese melts. Garnish with cilantro, if desired. Makes 4 servings.

Per serving: 265 calories; 11 g protein; 10 g fat; 35% calories from fat; 4 mg cholesterol; 32 g carbohydrates; 826 mg sodium; 3 g fiber

Chinese Eggplant and Scallion

1 large eggplant, stem removed and cut into 6 wedges
  water
2 tablespoons canola, corn, safflower, or sunflower oil
1 large green onion, cut into 2-inch pieces
2 tablespoons soy sauce
1/4 teaspoon sugar
  pepper to taste

In large skillet or Dutch oven, cook eggplant over medium heat in steamer basket or on rack over boiling water, 20 to 30 minutes or until tender. Heat oil in large skillet or wok over medium-high heat. Add green onion. Cook, stirring constantly, 1/2 minute. Add eggplant, soy sauce, sugar, and pepper. Cook, stirring constantly, 3 minutes or until heated through and well blended. Makes 4 servings.

Per serving: 113 calories; 2 g protein; 7 g fat; 51% calories from fat; 0 mg cholesterol; 12 g carbohydrates; 522 mg sodium; 6 g fiber

Delectable Desserts

Strawberry-Pineapple Crisp

12   ounces fresh strawberries (about 2 cups), sliced in half
1/2   fresh pineapple (about 3 1/2 pounds), peeled, cored,
        and cut into 1/2-inch cubes (about 3 cups)
6   tablespoons firmly packed brown sugar, divided
2   tablespoons cornstarch
1 1/4 cups unsweetened pineapple juice
1/2   cup regular or quick-cooking rolled oats
2   tablespoons all-purpose flour
2   tablespoons butter
1/2   teaspoon ground cinnamon

Preheat oven to 350°F. In greased 9-inch square baking dish, deep pie plate, or shallow 9-inch round casserole, gently toss strawberries and pineapple until well blended; set aside. In small saucepan, mix 2 tablespoons brown sugar with cornstarch. Stir in pineapple juice. Cook over medium heat, stirring constantly, 3 to 5 minutes or until thickened. Pour over fruit. In small bowl, stir remaining 1/4 cup brown sugar, oats, and flour. With fingers or pastry blender, cut in butter until mixture is crumbly; sprinkle evenly over strawberry-pineapple mixture. Top with cinnamon. Bake 30 to 35 minutes or until bubbly around edges and top is lightly browned. Makes 6 servings.

Per serving: 214 calories; 2 g protein; 5 g fat; 20% calories from fat; 10 mg cholesterol; 43 g carbohydrates; 41 mg sodium; 3.5 g fiber

Chocolate-Banana Thick Shake

2 medium very ripe bananas, cut into pieces
2½ cups skim milk, divided
2 tablespoons unsweetened cocoa powder
2 tablespoons sugar
1 cup fat-free chocolate ice cream

Place bananas, 1 cup skim milk, cocoa powder, and sugar in blender. Process until smooth. Add remaining skim milk and ice cream. Process until thick and foamy. Makes 4 servings.

Per serving: 180 calories; 9 g protein; 3 g fat; 13% calories from fat; 7 mg cholesterol; 33 g carbohydrates; 122 mg sodium; 2 g fiber

Lemon Glazed Tangerines

1   large lemon
1   large orange
    water
1/3 cup sugar
4   seedless tangerines or clementines, peeled
    and segmented

With zester or vegetable peeler, remove peel from lemon and orange (avoid the bitter white pith); reserve peels. Squeeze lemon; reserve juice. Save orange for another use. In small saucepan over high heat, bring to boil reserved lemon and orange peels and enough water to cover. Remove from heat; let stand 5 minutes. Drain. In same small saucepan, place drained peels, lemon juice, 1/2 cup water, and sugar. Bring to boil over medium-high heat. Reduce heat to low; simmer, uncovered, 10 to 15 minutes or until consistency of syrup. Cool, then strain. To serve, place tangerine segments in serving bowl; top with syrup. Toss to coat evenly. Chill 1 to 2 hours. Makes 4 servings.

Per serving: 94 calories; .5 g protein; .5 g fat; 1% calories from fat; 0 mg cholesterol; 24 g carbohydrates; 1 mg sodium; 2 g fiber

Cantaloupe-Strawberry Alaska

½ cup fresh strawberries, divided
1 small cantaloupe (about 1 pound), seeded and
   cut in half
2 tablespoons sweet sherry
¼ cup plus 2 teaspoons sugar, divided
2 egg whites, at room temperature
   pinch salt

Place ¼ cup strawberries into each cantaloupe half. Sprinkle strawberries evenly with sherry and 2 teaspoons sugar. Cover and chill at least 1 hour. Preheat oven to 400°F. To make meringue: In small bowl with mixer at high speed, beat egg whites until foamy. Gradually beat in remaining ¼ cup sugar until sugar is dissolved and stiff peaks form. Spoon ¼ whites evenly over each melon half. Place on baking sheet. Bake 5 minutes or until meringue is golden brown. Makes 2 servings.

Per serving: 160 calories; 4 g protein; .5 g fat; 4% calories from fat; 0 mg cholesterol; 36 g carbohydrates; 46 mg sodium; 3 g fiber

Strawberry-Yogurt Treat

1   cup fresh or frozen (thawed) strawberries
1   container (8 ounces) nonfat vanilla yogurt
1   cup club soda

Place all ingredients in blender and process until smooth. Makes 2 servings.

Per serving: 86 calories; 7 g protein; .5 g fat; 5% calories from fat; 2 mg cholesterol; 14 g carbohydrates; 112 mg sodium; 2 g fiber

Peachy-Almond Ice Milk

1 cup skim milk
2 tablespoons instant nonfat dry-milk powder
   fat-free, cholesterol-free egg substitute,
      equivalent to 1 egg
1/3 cup sugar
2 tablespoons amaretto liqueur (optional)
1 teaspoon vanilla extract
1/2 teaspoon almond extract
2 cups fresh (peeled) or frozen (thawed) sliced peaches
1 tablespoon lemon juice

To make custard: In medium saucepan over medium heat cook skim milk, milk powder, egg substitute, and sugar, stirring constantly, 5 to 8 minutes or until mixture is slightly thickened. Remove from heat; cover and chill at least 1 hour or until cool. Stir in liqueur and vanilla and almond extracts. In food processor or blender, puree peaches until smooth. Stir pureed peaches and lemon juice into cool custard. Freeze in ice cream maker according to manufacturer's directions or spoon into shallow metal baking pan and freeze, uncovered, until almost firm. Remove from pan and place in large bowl; beat peach mixture with mixer until slushy; return to chilled pan. Freeze until firm. Scoop and serve immediately. Makes 8 servings.

Note: Canned peaches may be used in the winter.

Per serving: 63 calories; 2 g protein; .5 g fat; 1% calories from fat; 0 mg cholesterol; 34 mg sodium; .5 g fiber

Blueberry and Pudding Parfait

1   cup fresh or frozen (thawed) unsweetened blueberries
2   tablespoons grape jelly
1   teaspoon sugar
1   teaspoon cornstarch mixed with 2 teaspoons water
1   package (4-serving size) cook-and-serve vanilla
      pudding-and-pie-filling mix
2   cups skim milk

Place blueberries and grape jelly into food processor or blender. Process until smooth. In small saucepan over medium heat, bring to boil, stirring constantly, blueberry-grape puree, sugar, and cornstarch mixture. Cook 1 minute more, stirring constantly. Remove from heat; let cool slightly. Cover and chill at least 30 minutes or until thickened. Prepare pudding according to package directions using skim milk; cool until just thickened. In each of four 6-ounce parfait glasses, layer 1/4 pudding and then 1/4 blueberry mixture, making alternate layers and ending with pudding. Cover and chill at least 1 hour or until set. Makes 4 servings.

Per serving: 114 calories; 4 g protein; .5 g fat; 3% calories from fat; 2 mg cholesterol; 24 g carbohydrates; 101 mg sodium; 1 g fiber

Kiwi-Lemon Sorbet

1 cup water
1/2 cup sugar
1/2 cup light corn syrup
4 kiwis, pared and cut in half
5 teaspoons lemon juice
1/4 teaspoon grated lemon peel

In small saucepan over medium heat, stir water, sugar, and corn syrup. Cook, stirring occasionally, 2 minutes or until sugar is dissolved. In food processor or blender, puree kiwis until smooth. Measure out 3/4 cup. (Save any remaining puree for another use.) In shallow metal baking pan, combine pureed kiwis, sugar syrup, lemon juice, and peel; freeze, uncovered, until almost firm. Remove and place in large bowl; beat kiwi mixture with mixer until light and fluffy; return to chilled baking pan. Freeze about 2 hours or until firm. Scoop and serve immediately. Makes 4 servings.

Per serving: 258 calories; 0 g protein; .5 g fat; 1% calories from fat; 0 mg cholesterol; 67 g carbohydrates; 23 mg sodium; 3 g fiber

Fruity Orange-Sicles

1   envelope unflavored gelatin
1/2 cup water
4   cups orange juice, divided
1/3 cup honey
1/2 cup pureed cantaloupe or peaches
10 5-ounce paper drinking cups

In medium saucepan, sprinkle gelatin over water; let stand 5 minutes or until softened. Stir in 1 cup orange juice and honey. Cook, stirring occasionally, 2 to 3 minutes or until gelatin dissolves. Stir in remaining orange juice and pureed fruit. Place ten 5-ounce paper drinking cups on tray or shallow baking pan. Fill with orange gelatin mixture almost to top and cover tray with foil. Insert wooden stick or plastic spoon in small hole in center of each cup. Freeze 3 hours or until firm. To serve, run warm water over outside and remove paper cup. Makes 10 servings.

Note: For longer storage, store in freezer, once frozen, in tightly closed plastic bag.

Per serving: 81 calories; 2 g protein; .5 g fat; 3% calories from fat; 0 mg cholesterol; 19 g carbohydrates; 3 mg sodium; 0 g fiber

No Bake Blueberry-Peach Pie

Crust
1   cup reduced-fat chocolate-wafer cookie crumbs
    (about 35 1-inch cookies)
2   tablespoons butter, melted
2   tablespoons honey

Filling
2   cups fresh or 1 package (12 ounces) frozen (thawed)
    blueberries, divided
1/4 cup water
1/4 cup sugar
2   tablespoons cornstarch
1 1/2 cups fresh, drained canned or frozen (thawed)
    sliced peaches
1   teaspoon vanilla extract

Preheat oven to 350°F. In medium bowl, mix chocolate cookie crumbs, butter, and honey until well blended. Press crumb mixture evenly on bottom and sides of 9-inch pie plate. Bake 8 to 10 minutes or until set and edges slightly brown. Remove from oven. Meanwhile, in medium saucepan over medium heat stir 1 cup blueberries, water, sugar, and cornstarch until well blended. Cook, stirring constantly, until mixture comes to boil. Boil, stirring constantly, 1 minute. Stir in remaining blueberries, peaches, and vanilla. Spoon into prepared crust. Chill at least 2 hours or until set. Makes 8 servings.

Per serving: 168 calories; 1 g protein; 4 g fat; 21% calories from fat; 8 mg cholesterol; 33 g carbohydrates; 92 mg sodium; 1.5 g fiber

CONVERSIONS

Metric Volume Equivalents

Measuring Cup			**Tablespoon**			**Teaspoon**		
1/4 cup	=	60 mL	1T	=	15 mL	1/4 t	=	1mL
1/3 cup	=	75 mL	2T	=	30 mL	1/2 t	=	2mL
1/2 cup	=	125 mL	3T	=	45 mL	1 t	=	5mL
3/4 cup	=	180 mL	4T	=	60 mL	2 t	=	10mL
1 cup	=	250 mL				3 t	=	15mL
2 cups	=	500 mL				4 t	=	20mL
3 cups	=	750 mL						
4 cup	=	1,000 mL						

Metric Weight Equivalents

1 ounce	=	30g
4 ounces (1/4 lb)	=	120g
12 ounces (3/4 lb)	=	225g
16 ounces (1 lb)	=	360g
32 ounces (2 lb)	=	900g

Oven Temperature Equivalents

Fahrenheit		Celsius
225°	=	110°
250°	=	120°
275°	=	140°
300°	=	150°
325°	=	160°
350°	=	180°
375°	=	190°
400°	=	200°
425°	=	220°